Your Journey to New Health

Lifestyle Approaches to Address Chronic Health Conditions

Your Journey to New Health

Lifestyle Approaches to Address Chronic Health Conditions

Donna Kay Jennings,
BSN, MHSA, MSN, PMHNP-BC

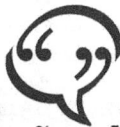

YouSpeakIt
PUBLISHING
The Easy Way
to Get Your Book
Done Right ™

www.YouSpeakItPublishing.com

ISBN: 978-1-945446-51-1

I dedicate this book to my new husband who, at age seventy-two, has reluctantly, but with good humor, started making changes to his lifestyle so that we can live a long, loving, healthy life together.

Acknowledgments

To Bryan Chalmers, my COO, who helped protect my time so that I could dedicate the many hours needed to research and write this book.

To my daughter and operations manager, Rosie Jennings, who has removed many burdens from me, and encouraged me to write this book.

To Dr. Chris Kresser, who has taught me through the ADAPT program to apply all of the information I learned from the Institute of Functional Medicine to my patients.

To Dr. David Elliot, who has spent many hours these past years reviewing labs and teaching me to be a better practitioner.

To my patients, who have good-naturedly gone along with my nontraditional approach to treating their complex chronic diseases, and to the many patients who have successfully changed their lives by changing their diet and lifestyle: You are truly my inspiration.

Contents

Introduction

Are you ready to make the journey to good health?

Ironically, this journey is often postponed until your health dictates that a change be made. The road can be littered with misinformation, old thinking, poor ideas, popular myths, and propaganda. The purpose of this book is to share the latest research-based ideas on health and wellness and to give practical solutions that can help you completely restore your health in only twelve months.

Sound too good to be true?

In this book, I break the journey into achievable goals, and I show you how to make lifestyle modifications that are practical, realistic, and effective.

I found myself in poor health at age fifty-five. I had high cholesterol, elevated blood sugar, and insomnia. I was on medications for each of these conditions. I was overweight; in fact, without realizing it, I had actually slid into obesity. I had recently completed schooling to become an APRN (Advanced Practice Registered Nurse) and preparing for the national boards had stressed me to the point of having a severe case of shingles.

My first day of seeing patients as a newly licensed nurse practitioner ended with chest pain and an overnight stay at the hospital. I felt exhausted and overwhelmed. This situation pushed me into a journey to find a way to cure my body and restore my health. The quest for recovery led me to a wonderful new field of medicine.

The human body has an amazing ability to maintain its own health, and if insulted or damaged, to repair itself. When harmful signals are removed and the appropriate messages are delivered to the cells, the healthy body can be restored. Healthcare professionals can assist in this process.

This kind of approach may have many different names.

Some of them are listed below:

- Lifestyle therapy
- Holistic approach
- Alternative medicine
- Ancestral health
- Functional medicine

My personal quest for recovery led me to the wonderful field of *integrative functional medicine,* and this has become my approach to medicine and healthcare. I was a healthcare professional who was well trained in the traditional *allopathic* model of care, but I've crossed over to a very different model.

What is the difference?

Allopathic medicine is considered to be mainstream, Western, or traditional medicine. Allopathic healthcare practitioners will generally treat your symptoms with pharmaceuticals or surgery. Functional medicine practitioners consider your symptoms but determine the root cause and thus get a more permanent solution using lifestyle interventions. The practice of integrative functional medicine relies on the amazing ability of the body to heal itself, instead of relying on the pharmaceutical industry.

Imagine that your automobile's check engine light comes on. You take the car in to the mechanic. They reset the light, but never look under the hood to see what the root cause is. You drive off, only to have the light come on again the next day. You go back into the mechanic. They reset the light, but again, they neglect to look under the hood.

How many times do you keep going back to have the light reset?

Now, compare this to a woman who feels like there's something wrong with her. Her eyebrows have thinned, her hair is falling out, she has little energy, she's somewhat depressed, her sleep is poor, and her skin is dry. She goes to her doctor, who tests for thyroid dysfunction with a simple TSH (thyroid stimulating hormone) test, which turns out to be within the normal range. Her doctor, of course, tells her she's fine. She returns the following year feeling worse and is given the same test. The results are, again, within normal range.

What does her doctor do now?

Many doctors, thinking it must all be in her head, would give her an antidepressant.

If this same woman had gone to a functional medicine practitioner, seven or eight lab tests would have been ordered, the lab range would have been narrower, and the root cause of her thyroid symptoms would have been discovered. This condition would have been treated with diet, exercise, and proper support at the cellular level.

The practice of functional medicine is shifting from a disease focus to a focus on the patient, shifting from covering up symptoms with medications to finding the root cause for those symptoms.

As a functional medicine practitioner, I consider:

- Environmental causes
- Genetics
- Inflammation
- Immune system
- Lifestyle and diet

I also get to know you as an individual and learn what your stressors are.

Functional medicine uses philosophies that have been around for a long time. Given the state of health in this century, it is especially useful right now. Methods such as these were employed by Hippocrates himself 2,500 years ago.

The Institute of Functional Medicine (IFM) teaches that there is also a huge gap between research and the way doctors' practice. The gap between emerging research and the implementation of this research into practice is enormous — as long as fifteen years. IFM also asserts in multiple lectures that most physicians are not adequately trained to assess the underlying cause of chronic complex disease, and to apply strategies such as nutrition, diet, and exercise to both treat and prevent these diseases.

Functional medicine is different from allopathic medicine in several ways:

1. It is *patient-centered.* It embraces the idea that health is not just the absence of disease but also living a life with health and vitality.

2. Functional medicine relies very strongly on an *integrative, science-based approach.*

3. It integrates traditional Western medical practices with what are sometimes called *alternative* approaches, using the latest in lab testing, diagnostic techniques, prescriptions of combined botanical medicine supplements, therapeutic diet and detoxification programs, and stress management techniques.

Functional medicine practitioners empower patients by teaching them what the root cause is and equipping them with the knowledge to live a vital life.

CHAPTER ONE

The Five Rs—Remove, Replace, Reinoculate, Repair, Rebalance

INFLAMMATION

During my years working in functional medicine healthcare, I have come to understand that most chronic health conditions are related to inflammation. We have a very inflamed society.

Why is inflammation so commonplace?

Here are the major factors that contribute to inflammation:

- Diet
- Lack of exercise
- Toxins
- Trauma
- Bugs — meaning microbial pathogens
- Environmental triggers

I have learned that inflammation is at the root of most chronic diseases. If you can identify what the source of the inflammation is, then you can treat the condition.

What Is Inflammation?

As we go through life, we encounter various viruses, bacteria, toxins, and fungi that attack our body. Our bodies are uniquely designed to fight these invaders, whether it's a wooden splinter, a bacterium, or a virus. You have an immune system that will respond to any insult to your body. When your system is balanced, you're healthy. This means you have a healthy immune system that can effectively fight any invaders.

If you have a bacterial infection, for instance, a healthy immune system can fight the bacterial infection and go back to a balanced state. If you don't have a healthy immune system, however, you can become chronically inflamed, and that triggers disease. It's as simple as a teeter-totter. You either have a healthy biological system, or you have an unhealthy system—and the unhealthy system leads to chronic disease.

When you have stressors, like bugs, trauma, toxins, and stress—and it's important to realize that stress itself is damaging to your body—they trigger the immune system in your intestines. Your intestines will respond to these stressors in a way that results in inflammation.

This inflammation can affect your whole gut—the small intestine, large intestine, and stomach.

This inflammation can start to penetrate the protective barriers in your body and allow foreign proteins, bacterial toxins, and food particles through. Your immune system then sets up an attack against these foreign particles, causing allergic responses and autoimmune responses.

The imbalance that is caused by inflammation in your gut can cause many different problems:

- Allergies
- Asthma
- Thyroid dysfunction
- Autoimmune disease, like Hashimoto's
- Nerve disease, like Guillain-Barré syndrome
- Depression
- Mental health issues
- Chronic fatigue

Inflammation is one of our defense mechanisms. Under normal conditions, if you become inflamed, that's your body trying to heal itself. If you get a cut that gets a little bit infected, it will become inflamed as your immune system reacts and responds appropriately. The inflammatory process helps the immune system to clean up the area and prepare it so that the wound can heal.

Inflammation in itself is not bad. I don't want people to think inflammation is bad, because it isn't—when it's in a normal, healthy body. However, if your body is imbalanced and you develop inflammation in your organs and tissues, it will have a damaging effect. Dr. Dale Bredesen states that there is a direct mechanistic link between inflammation and Alzheimer's disease.[1] Although it will likely be debated for the next fifteen years, most nonpharmaceutical research agrees that there is a strong association between inflammation and Alzheimer's.

People need to get serious about chronic inflammation because it can have an impact on all the tissues and organs of the body. Inflammation was designed to protect us from injuries and bacteria; it was not designed to be a chronic condition.

Assessing and Diagnosing Inflammation

Lots of different kinds of folks come to my practice.

What brings them in?

Here are the most common complaints:

- Fatigue
- Obesity

---

1   Bredesen, Dale. *The End of Alzheimer's*. Avery Publishing, 2017.

- Mind not working well
- Simply not feeling well

As you can see, generally, these symptoms are not very specific.

When they come into the practice, most people look relatively healthy. If you were to estimate health by visual assessment, you might say some look a little overweight, or they seem like they're dragging a little bit, but generally, they look as though they are okay.

If these patients go to a traditional allopathic practitioner, here is what would most likely happen:

- If the patient were overweight, they would be told: *Eat less, move more.*

- They wouldn't have any testing done for obesity, except for a blood glucose test.

- If the patient came in with fatigue, the practitioner might run a standard blood count (CBC) to check for anemia, although a CBC in itself wouldn't test for the full source of anemia.

- It is very unlikely the practitioner would assess the condition of the gut; rarely would they run a stool specimen.

- Tests to check inflammation would rarely be ordered.

- Only basic tests would be performed, and they would likely come back normal, so the person going into a traditional practitioner would get the response: *There's nothing wrong with you. Your labs are all fine.*

In conclusion, if you were this patient, you would most likely be sent home with no answers, and your symptoms would continue.

What would happen if you went back to that doctor again with the same symptoms?

When a patient revisits repeatedly with vague symptoms, many traditionally trained physicians will determine that the patient is probably just depressed, and they will begin treatment for depression.

I have a background in psychiatry, and I am sorry to say that I see this far too often. Lots of folks who come see me have already been given an antidepressant from their primary care doctor simply because they have persistent vague symptoms. Instead of getting down to the root cause, they get a pill.

A Different Way

In contrast, I do a full workup on each patient who comes through my door.

We collect samples and seek results from:

- A full blood workup
- Stool analysis
- Adrenal testing

I run these basic tests for everyone. I'm starting to add some genetic testing as well, to help me know who is predisposed to what. If a patient shows a predisposition to a chronic illness, it's more important than ever to minimize inflammation.

We check the functioning of the gut and do assessments for inflammation. Internal inflammation is not apparent on the outside; testing is required. Patients usually have no idea how inflamed they are until they see the results of their tests.

When I do the blood work, I look at *C Reactive Protein* (CRP), which is one of the main indicators of inflammation. Blood levels of this protein rise with inflammation. *Homocysteine* is another inflammatory marker, and there are others as well. These indicators tell us whether inflammation exists, but they don't tell us the source of inflammation in the body.

We must start an investigative process to figure out what is the root cause of their symptoms. That's generally what leads us to figure out what is causing inflammation. For example, we run a stool specimen, and that stool specimen indicates whether the patient has a fungal overgrowth, like a yeast overgrowth. Or, we may discover that there is a bacterial infection, or the patient may have a *dysbiosis* of the gut—an imbalance in the naturally occurring bacteria in the gut.

Treatment: The Five R Framework

In functional medicine, we always look to the gut first. We'll discuss this in more detail in a later section of the book. Even though patients may not have symptoms of a gut disorder, many have something going in in their gut that is causing problems. Many people we test have either an *intestinal permeability,* which in layman's terms we call *leaky gut,* or they have dysbiosis. Sometimes, a patient has a *small intestine bacterial overgrowth* (SIBO).

To restore a patient back to health, we always use the *Five R Framework* for gut restoration.

The Five R Framework, which was developed by the Institute for Functional Medicine (IFM) consists of these five pillars of treatment:

- Remove
- Replace
- Reinoculate
- Repair
- Rebalance

No matter the cause, this framework can always be used. If we restore the gut, we can restore the patient to health.

The First R: *Remove*

What do we need to remove?

- Stressors
- Foods that the patient might be allergic or sensitive to
- Parasites
- Nonbeneficial Bacteria
- Fungi or yeast
- Anything else that is negatively impacting the gut

On the first visit with a new patient, before I even know what's wrong with them, I start them on an elimination diet while I'm waiting for the various test results to come back. The elimination diet involves removing foods that most people have a sensitivity to. We remove the top five or six foods in their diet that are likely culprits.

Commonly, this will include some of these items:

- Coffee
- Alcohol
- Sugar

- Gluten
- Some of the nightshades, like tomatoes

For a full description of the diet, please see the appendix.

The Second R: *Replace*

Due to diet, medications, aging, or other factors, there are often critical digestive secretions missing from the gut of the patient, like digestive enzymes, hydrochloric acid, and bile salts. We assess the gut and devise a strategy to replace missing elements that are required for proper digestion.

The Third R: *Reinoculate*

Reinoculating helps the beneficial bacteria flourish. We always offer a high-potency variety of *probiotics* to patients. Probiotics are friendly bacteria that help the gut to rid itself of bad bacteria. We teach people how to make their own fermented sauerkraut and their own bone broth. We show them easy and inexpensive ways to restore health to their gut.

Foods that feed the probiotics are called *prebiotics*.

Some examples of prebiotics are:

- Artichokes
- Garlic

- Leeks
- Onions
- Chicory
- Tofu
- Grains, such as barley and oats

The Fourth R: *Repair*

Many chronic inflammatory conditions result in damage to the mucosal lining in the gut. There may be a permeability problem or leaky gut or immune upregulation. Repair is necessary to replenish the building blocks in the body so healing can take place.

I use a combination of botanicals and other natural factors to promote repair of the lining of the gut. Often, when you combine certain natural healing ingredients in specific proportions, you get more of an effect than you would get separately. They usually are available to practitioners in combinations.

Many different factors can assist with gut repair, but some of the key ingredients are:

- Zinc
- Antioxidants
- A, C, and E vitamins
- Fish oil
- Amino acids
- Glutamine

Note that patients should not just go out and buy these off the shelf; you really need to go to a reliable practitioner to get good products in the correct proportions.

The Fifth R: *Rebalance*

We take a holistic approach to gut restoration. In order to restore health, you have to assess the root causes of the imbalance. Only then can you can genuinely return to a balanced state.

What caused your gut to get out of balance in the first place?

What was the trigger?

To find the root causes, we need to get to know the patient. We look at the whole person: their lifestyle, their habits, and their timeline, from birth to their current age.

When you see a functional practitioner, you would be asked questions like these:

- What is your lifestyle like?

- What important events have occurred in your life?

- Have you used antibiotics frequently?

- What are your dietary habits?

- Do you drink many sodas or cups of coffee a day?

- How well do you sleep?

- What is your stress level?

- What kind of exercise do you get?

An essential feature of functional medicine is looking at everything that impacts the patient's health. With each patient who has chronic inflammation, we work on rebalancing whatever is going on in that person's life, with the understanding that it all affects the gastrointestinal (GI) tract, as well as the rest of the body.

THE IMMUNE SYSTEM

The immune system is a complex system that requires a great deal of study. I have a multitude of books on this one system.

What is the immune system and how does it work?

Your immune system is a natural defense system that helps fight infection. It's made up of white blood cells, antibodies, and chemicals that attack and destroy substances—such as bacteria or viruses—that it recognizes as foreign.

Your immune system, which has adapted and matured since infancy, is designed to recognize and respond to any foreign invader. Imagine your body is like a house that someone is trying to break into. The immune system is activated when something unfamiliar makes its way through the natural outer barriers, like your skin and mucosal barriers.

The immune system includes a diverse collection of cells and tissues, including:

- Glands, like the tonsils and the thymus
- Lymphocytes or white blood cells
- The lymphatic system
- The spleen
- Bone marrow

Some parts of the immune system, including the tonsils and the thymus, make *antibodies,* which your immune system uses to neutralize pathogens. The *lymphatic system,* which is a network of lymph nodes and vessels, carries wastes out through lymph fluid, and it filters out and traps bacteria and viruses so they can be destroyed by the white blood cells. The bone marrow is a part of the lymphatic system as well. It creates many of the cells that make up the immune system. The spleen, which filters the blood by removing the damaged cells and platelets, also helps the immune system by destroying bacteria.

The white blood cells, made in the bone marrow, protect the body against infection. Any time you have a CBC done, a white blood cell count is taken and this count helps us know if you have an infection. Your body produces more pathogen-fighting white blood cells when it detects an invader. Therefore, your white blood cell count is elevated when an infection is present. In addition, the levels of other cells in your blood will change based on the level of inflammation.

What Is an Autoimmune Disorder?

In my functional medicine practice, I have been overwhelmed by the sheer number of people who come in telling me they *just don't feel well.* Most of them have already had a doctor look at their basic labs.

I do some antibody testing when these patients come in, including a test for antibodies in the thyroid. The thyroid is integral; every cell in your body needs the thyroid hormone *triiodothyronine* (T3). If you're not making or converting thyroid hormone, then you have a problem, and for a lot of people, it presents as fatigue and weight gain. I always check the thyroid thoroughly. A traditional doctor will most likely only test for TSH, which often doesn't help with diagnosis on its own. In contrast, I do eight or nine tests for the thyroid, including assessing antibodies.

The antibodies tell me if the immune system is overreacting. Often, I find that people with vague symptoms have an autoimmune disorder of their thyroid gland, one of which is called *Hashimoto's disease* (autoimmune thyroiditis). Sometimes, I can identify Hashimoto's before a patient starts showing changes in their TSH levels, simply by noticing elevated levels of antibodies. Sixty percent of women with a thyroid disorder have Hashimoto's, and we can identify the presence of this autoimmune disorder early by choosing the right tests to run.

When someone has an autoimmune disorder, the immune system is overreacting to something that has gotten into the bloodstream, usually from the gut— from a leaky gut—and has started producing antibodies to a part of your own body.

In the case of Hashimoto's disease, the immune system produces antibodies to receptors in the thyroid gland, and as a result, the immune system starts attacking the thyroid gland.

Studying the immune system is important, because many diseases have an autoimmune factor to them. More than two hundred diseases are connected to autoimmunity.

Here are a few:

- Arthritis
- Ankylosing spondylitis
- Systemic lupus erythematosus
- Reiter's syndrome
- Autoimmune hepatitis
- Sjögren's syndrome
- Type 1 diabetes
- Scleroderma
- Dermatomyositis
- Hashimoto's disease
- Rheumatoid arthritis
- Multiple sclerosis
- Grave's disease
- Autoimmune pancreatitis

If you are one of the many people who have an autoimmune disorder, if you can calm the immune system by removing the bugs, the trauma, the toxins — whatever is triggering the immune system — you can calm down the symptoms of the disease. If you can remove the triggers, you can keep the condition in remission. While you'll never get rid of the disorder, you can eliminate the symptoms.

How We Diagnose Autoimmune Disease

There are ways to check to see if an autoimmune disease exists; for example, we can test to see if the body is producing antibodies against certain proteins that characterize autoimmune conditions. If you have celiac disease, for instance, the autoimmunity is related to gluten. That's easy to pick up with a serum test.

Antibody testing is crucial. With it, you can pick up a wide variety of autoimmune issues, from gluten sensitivity to rheumatoid arthritis. In my practice, we send serum samples to the lab based on the symptoms of the patient. The symptoms will lead you to suspect certain things that you can then verify with testing.

One other way that I rule out sensitivities that cause your immune system to go awry is by prescribing an elimination diet, as mentioned earlier. It's an inexpensive way to rule out foods that may be triggering symptoms, including autoimmunity.

If your symptoms clear up after you've eliminated a few things, you may have found your trigger. An elimination diet is crucial for anyone who doesn't feel well, and you can do it yourself. You can find directions for an elimination diet in the appendix of this book.

My advice is to start simply by eliminating the top foods, mentioned in the earlier section of this chapter, to see if your condition is caused by a food allergy or a food sensitivity.

How We Treat Autoimmune Disease

An allopathic practitioner will likely put you on medications for an autoimmune disease. A lot of these medications are steroids, prescribed to keep the antibody level and the inflammation down. In contrast, in functional medicine, we generally go after whatever is triggering the inflammation and the immune system response, whether it is a toxin, bug, food, or other factor.

Autoimmune issues are most often caused by diet. The standard American diet is full of toxins, and they come in the form of preservatives in your food that give foods a longer shelf life, as well as in plastic linings and the jars and cans that hold food.

In addition to preservatives, other common triggers include:

- Trans fats
- Artificial sweeteners
- Food colorings

If you can go to a fresh-food diet, and eliminate processed and refined foods, your triggers may be eliminated.

Besides the toxins associated with our foods, toxins in the environment may function as triggers. Mold is a big one that triggers a lot of autoimmunity. You can get a test online to check your house for mold. Wipe your house down, send the cloth into the company, and they'll check for mold in your home. You have to eliminate all sources of mold in your home.

You may want to start drinking filtered water. You can learn the content of the water in your municipality if you go on the Environmental Work Group (EWG) website.[2] Not only do I filter my drinking water, which contains chlorine, but I also have to filter my shower water. You can inhale those toxins, and they can trigger autoimmunity like asthma. I do have asthma, and I have attributed some of my symptoms to my water source.

The EWG website is a great resource. The site also has information about the chemicals that are in your toiletries, cosmetics, and household cleaning products. You can investigate every product you use, and possibly find better ones.

Getting rid of toxins will go a long way to calm your immune system, so it doesn't have to work so hard to protect your body.

---

2   ewg.org

HOW WE ADDRESS CHRONIC HEALTH CONDITIONS

I've been a registered nurse since 1973. During the first thirty years of my career, I was working in a traditional allopathic setting. About ten years ago, I decided I would go back to school and become a nurse practitioner. I chose psychiatry as a specialty because I saw there was a huge need in this area. While the causes of death remain largely the same in the psychiatric population as in the typical population, the median reduction in life expectancy for people with mental illness worldwide is ten years, attributed to chronic co-morbid conditions.[3]

After I was awarded my psychiatry nurse practitioner degree, I started practicing functional psychiatry. I went to a lot of trainings, and that's when I really developed a passion for treating chronic health conditions.

After all, the brain is attached to the body, and so, when patients come in with a brain condition, we must also heal the body. I came to understand that if you don't heal the body, total remission from psychiatric problems is not possible. As my understanding has progressed, my passion — for treating all kinds of people — has grown and grown over the years.

---

3   Walker, E. R.; McGee, R. E.; and Druss, B. G. "Mortality in Mental Disorders and Global Disease Burden Implications." *JAMA Psychiatry.* 2015;72(4):334–341. DOI:10.1001/jamapsychiatry.2014.2502

In particular, I'm now focused on Alzheimer's prevention and reversal because that, too, is an inflammatory disease that can be treated. You treat it in the same way I've described. As I learned more about functional medicine, I got really excited about how simple and inexpensive it is to treat chronic health conditions functionally, versus the allopathic, traditional way in which you use pharmaceutical drugs — and which costs billions of dollars.

The Top Causes of Death

The Centers for Disease Control and Prevention (CDC) usually provides a list of the top causes of death each year. The positions on the list change from time to time and vary by age. On the CDC website, you can view the statistics in detail.[4] In this section, I'd like to discuss the diseases most commonly found near the top of the list.

If you discard accidents, which are generally third or fourth on the list, the list is generally like this:

1. Cardiovascular disease
2. Cancer
3. Respiratory conditions
4. Stroke
5. Alzheimer's
6. Diabetes

---

4   cdc.gov/injury/wisqars/LeadingCauses.html

We will discuss each of these below. Note that I've included strokes in the discussion of cardiovascular disease.

Cardiovascular Diseases and Strokes

Cardiovascular disease includes anything that affects the cardiovascular system—from hypertension to strokes to heart attacks.

When you consult with a traditional doctor and your blood pressure is a little elevated, the doctor will prescribe a blood pressure pill. When you go back in six months, and your blood pressure is still elevated, they'll give you a diuretic. When you go back in another year, you'll be prescribed a higher dosage or more medication.

There are a lot of side effects to blood pressure medications. For example, a lot of males don't like their blood pressure meds because a side effect is erectile dysfunction.

You will be told to reduce fats and cut cholesterol from your diet. One of the myths about cardiovascular disease is that you need to eliminate fat and cholesterol from your diet to improve cardiovascular health. Cholesterol is actually healthy for your brain and your body. Cholesterol is necessary for the successful function of many of your hormones, such as estrogen, testosterone, progesterone, aldosterone, and cortisone.

Inflammation in the vessels is what causes increases in blood pressure; so, once again, we have an inflammatory process going on. Traditional medicine doesn't address inflammation in the cardiovascular system, with one exception—some doctors advise patients to take aspirin, which does reduce inflammation.

In the functional medicine world, if you were to come in with hypertension, first and foremost we're going to figure out the status of the inflammatory markers. Then we will start an intensive investigation. We will look at *everything*.

We will ask:

- What's going on internally?
- What else is happening that's triggering inflammation?
- Are you drinking enough water?
- Are your kidneys working well?
- Are you overweight?
- How are you breathing at night?
- Are you having sleep apnea?
- What is your diet like?
- Do you exercise?
- What is your level of stress?

If you have sleep apnea, this can affect the cardiovascular system. About 60 percent of Americans have some type of sleep apnea, but many don't know it because it has not been diagnosed. We can send you home with a home test kit for a night, to check if you're experiencing sleep apnea at night.

As I've said, we talk about diet with all patients, including those with cardiovascular issues. We create a cardio-metabolic lifestyle plan, which gives you a list of nutritious foods that you can eat. We do not give you a list of foods that you *can't* eat; we just give you lots of choices of foods that you *can* eat. If you are overweight, we work with you on a plan to lose weight.

Then we monitor your blood pressure. We take three readings when you're sitting and relaxed; you really have to put in the time to get a completely accurate measurement. Then we recommend you purchase a home blood pressure cuff, so you can keep an eye on your blood pressure at home.

We start an exercise program, and we work on eliminating the foods that cause inflammation. We start fixing any nutritional deficiencies, if that is also an issue. We give you supplements that may help relax your cardiovascular system, such as magnesium, which is great for relaxing the musculoskeletal system, reducing muscle cramps, and contributing to better sleep.

Cancer

Cancer is inflammation embodied. Cancer is caused by inflammation, and cancers have pervasive inflammation as a side effect.

You may be predisposed to developing cancer, but everything we've been talking about — diet, bugs, and toxins in the environment — may contribute to cancer, depending on the type of cancer. We will discuss this more in a later chapter.

To reduce your risk of cancer, focus on:

- Early intervention, including preventive screenings, such as mammography and colonoscopy
- Knowing your risks
- Living a good and healthy lifestyle

Consider, for example, the number-one cancer: lung cancer. If you eliminate smoking, cigarettes, and tobacco products, and you try to stay away from a lot of fumes from automobiles, you will reduce your cancer risk.

When a traditional doctor finds cancer, an often-used strategy is to cut it out surgically. In my functional practice, we generally don't find cancer, but if we do, we refer the patient to an oncologist and focus our energies on helping the patient maintain the best possible health during cancer treatment.

Respiratory Conditions

The most common respiratory conditions are bronchitis, emphysema, asthma, and chronic obstructive pulmonary disease (COPD).

I had late-onset asthma at age sixty-five. I saw my doctor for my first appointment under Medicare and came out with a list of a hundred tests I needed to do. I found out that I have asthma, which is unusual at my age. Asthma, like many other respiratory conditions, is treated with inhalers, which are very expensive. Medicare pays for part, but you pay the rest of it out of your pocket.

A patient with asthma either gets put on oxygen or has to keep using these inhalers for the rest of their life. The cost of treating these diseases traditionally can be astronomical.

In functional medicine, we look at asthma as an immune system reaction to something, so we put our efforts into figuring out what toxin is causing the reaction and then, work on that. I know smoke triggers mine, and it was just exacerbated because of local forest fires. In the functional world, you figure out what's triggering the symptoms, and then you provide the appropriate support. There's a lot of nutritional, botanical support you can apply to help your lung tissues get stronger and healthier.

In the traditional world, for these chronic conditions like asthma, you would likely be told: *You're going to have this the rest of your life.*

In the functional world, we say: *Let's get your condition treated so it's under control, so that you won't have to use those inhalers and oxygen for the rest of your life*

Alzheimer's Disease

Cognitive decline and Alzheimer's disease has been, in the past, a death sentence. Even today, in many traditional medical practices, if you get that diagnosis, it would be considered a death sentence. You are going to die from the disease.

Many practitioners will give you a pill and tell you to come back in six months, but they are not likely to design a treatment plan focusing on reversal or improvement of symptoms.

Using functional medicine strategies, we know now that we can help. Our approaches have helped to fix and identify forty different errors that commonly occur in the brains of patients with Alzheimer's disease. We focus on the key drivers of cognitive decline, such as insulin resistance, inflammation, nutritional and hormonal deficiencies, and toxins.

The Alzheimer's brain has been compared to a roof with forty holes. In a traditional treatment, a drug will fill maybe one or two holes. The functional medicine approach goes after all of the forty holes in the roof instead, and we are having some exciting successes.

Dr. Dale Bredesen of the Buck Institute, UCLA, is one research neurologist who has been successfully reversing, healing, and preventing Alzheimer's. It is so exciting that functional medicine can do something for a disease that, up until now, has been seen as a death sentence.

Diabetes

Diabetes of all types is another leading cause of death.

You may have a genetic predisposition to type 1 diabetes, and if you do have this condition, lifestyle changes can help you manage it so you can minimize symptoms.

In traditional medicine, whether you have type 1 or type 2, you see your provider and get a medication, you get your little finger stick to check your glucose, and you are put on insulin. If you have type 2 diabetes, you're prescribed oral meds — sometimes multiple prescriptions — and eventually insulin.

You will be told to go see a nutritionist. The problem with that is most nutritionists are still operating under the old idea that these patients should be eating lots of grains — and this will not help people with their diabetes.

In contrast, we generally take them off all gluten, as well as all processed and refined foods, so that they eat only vegetables, proteins, and good fats. That tends to stabilize and reverse type 2 diabetes if we catch people early enough. We tend to catch them early in functional medicine because we do an A1C test, which tells us the patient's average blood sugar over a three-month period. In traditional medicine, this test is not done with your annual workup.

When we do an A1C, we can see what the average blood sugar is and if it is spiking. We also measure insulin to see if it is in the proper range. We are able to identify diabetes way before it hits, way before you can diagnose it, and we immediately start lifestyle interventions at that time. Functional medicine really can treat diabetes. It's just amazing what we can do for someone who is diabetic.

Obesity contributes to and increases the degree of risk for all types of diabetes. Obesity just makes everything worse; obesity in itself is inflammatory. When they follow the functional medicine protocol that we offer, most of our overweight patients lose a significant amount of weight. When we get people to change their lifestyle, they naturally take the excess weight off during the process.

Allopathic Training and Treatments

In this chapter, we've discussed the allopathic model of healthcare and its failures to treat patients effectively, when compared with treatment using functional medicine.

Why then, does the conventional medical training system continue to follow the same kind of curriculum, when it is clearly outdated?

We know that students go to medical school to become doctors because they want to help people; they are not lacking in motivation.

The fact that these medical schools are largely funded by the pharmaceutical industry may give us part of the answer, for this fact may strongly affect the curriculum. When I trained as a nurse practitioner, I was trained to treat symptoms for any medical condition with a medication. I came to object to this approach because I didn't see good outcomes.

In the allopathic, traditional model, when a patient walks in with a symptom, they are most likely treated with some medication. If it doesn't get better, another medication is added. This is largely what's contributing to the rising prices in healthcare; medications are extremely expensive.

Most practitioners get a lot of their education from the drug companies, and when doctors go to conferences, guess who the sponsors are?

The sponsors are the drug companies.

Medical tradition provides standard algorithms that guide the doctor in what to do—or in what drug to prescribe. That's traditional medicine.

The Functional Approach

In functional medicine, on the other hand, we treat all these conditions functionally.

What does this mean?

We take all of their symptoms and look at them in groupings. We try to figure out which organ—or organs—are involved. Then we do a full spread of tests. We do way more testing than a traditional practitioner typically does. We do very thorough lab testing, including blood, stool, genes, and more, and then we start at the root: we search for the root cause and start treatment there.

After testing the patient thoroughly, we review the symptoms and the test results from a whole-body perspective. We understand that all of the body is fully connected — the brain, the gut, all the organs and systems. It's all connected.

Every patient's care is individualized, and each patient has a different treatment plan, based on the root cause of their symptoms and their particular circumstances. It's not by the book, not by an algorithm. It is based completely on the needs of that individual patient.

CHAPTER TWO

Exercise, Energy, Sleep, and Stress Management

HOW TO IDENTIFY AND MANAGE STRESS

Stress affects all of us, especially in modern society. Learning how to deal with that stress effectively can have a huge impact on our body, and our ability to recover and to live a healthy life. I think we need to find new ways to address stress in our society because our bodies were originally designed to respond to stress thousands of years ago, when lives were very different. When a lion appeared, for example, our bodies responded with a stress response, which starts in the sympathetic nervous system. Today, that same stress response does not serve us as well as it did when we were running through the forest.

The Physiological Effects of Stress

One of the best books that I have read on stress is *Why Zebras Don't Get Ulcers* by Robert Sapolsky (Holt Paperbacks, 2004). It's an excellent book for people who want to know more about stress and how we deal with it.

To understand how stress affects the body, you need to understand the adrenal glands. In a nutshell, the adrenal glands, which sit on top of the kidneys, respond to stress by secreting adrenaline to give you a boost of energy. They also secrete cortisol in response to stress.

Cortisol regulates many body systems, such as:

- Blood sugar
- Macronutrient metabolism
- Immune response
- Anti-inflammatory response
- Cardiovascular tone
- Blood pressure
- Central nervous system activation

When stress becomes chronic, the adrenals sometimes can't keep up with the demand. These glands can actually become exhausted, causing them to work inadequately. In addition, when you over-secrete adrenaline, this can cause you to feel anxious and nervous.

Too much adrenaline causes complaints of:

- Insomnia
- Fatigue
- Depression
- Irritability

Too much adrenaline can cause a variety of digestive difficulties as well.

In the long-term, chronically high cortisol and adrenaline can cause:

- Diminished immune function
- Low blood sugar, due to depletion of cortisol
- Less restful sleep
- Increased blood pressure
- Water retention
- Electrolyte imbalances
- Diminished insulin sensitivity, which can contribute to diabetes
- Loss of capacity to produce sufficient dehydroepiandrosterone (DHEA)

DHEA is another important hormone produced by the adrenal glands. Insufficient amounts of this hormone can affect health in several ways.

Under normal circumstances, DHEA:

- Helps to make both testosterone and estrogen

- Improves resistance to viruses, bacteria, parasites, allergies, and cancers
- Helps prevent osteoporosis
- Lowers your total LDL cholesterol
- Increases muscle mass and decreases body fat

You can see how stress can impact body weight indirectly if it causes diminished levels of DHEA. Many Americans—30 percent or more—are overweight to morbidly obese. It's a critical problem, and it greatly affects health issues.

Diagnosing Stress

In my practice, I regularly see patients for a functional medicine review and workup. I always ask questions about stress. The majority of people will say that they don't have stressors in their lives, but when their adrenal tests come back, I can tell that they are under stress. Together, we have to look more closely at their lives to see how they manage stress. Most people don't realize that stress is so critical to their overall health.

I look at these critical elements when I am assessing stress:

- Blood sugar
- Potential causes of stress in the patient, and measurement of stress level
- Sleep disturbances

- Inflammation
- Adrenal function
- Thyroid function

The first area that I look at is *blood sugar*. If the blood sugar is imbalanced — if they have a high blood sugar or a high insulin level — I know that they're not managing stress well. Stress affects blood sugar.

Second, we need to identify *what is causing stress*. There are different kinds of stress and the list of things that contribute to stress is huge. For mental and emotional stress, there are several scales to address your stress level. I think the top one is loss, or death of a loved one. The second one is bankruptcy. You need to identify which ones are affecting you.

Third, if a patient tells me they have a *sleep disturbance,* again I know that they are going through stress, because you should sleep well if you're not stressed. Sleep is critical to managing stress.

Fourth, I look for *inflammation*. Any type of inflammation has a stress component — whether you have a gut problem, suffer from headaches, muscle aches or pains, dermatological hives, psoriasis, respiratory problems, such as asthma or bronchitis, or any autoimmune or immunological problems, such as chronic infections and frequent illnesses. If a patient has one of these conditions, we know we will be diving deeply into an investigation of stress.

Fifth, we look at the *functioning of the thyroid*. When I'm diagnosing stress, I always look at hormone levels to see how the thyroid is doing. Many people don't realize that stress may play an important role in thyroid dysfunction. There is a relationship between the adrenals and how well your thyroid functions. Chronic stress and inflammation increase the body's demand for cortisol, and high levels of cortisol directly suppress thyroid function. It's critical for your cells to have T3 in them, and high levels of cortisol prevent the thyroid hormone T4 *(thyroxine)* from converting to T3. It's crucial that we address the thyroid when assessing how the body is functioning. To do this, I assess thyroid hormone levels.

Stress-Management Techniques

If you came into our practice, and we found that your adrenals were not operating optimally, or you had another marker that indicates the need for stress management, we would proceed to work on stress.

We would have to identify your stressors; we would be looking for the root causes. Remember, that's what functional medicine is — looking at the root causes of everything — and this includes stress.

Most people think stressors are emotional alone in nature, but physical stressors contribute a lot. It could be that you're not managing your blood sugar, or you have an infection, or there's something else going on in your body. We will examine your whole body to identify any physical stressors so that we can treat them.

For emotional stressors, here are some stress-management suggestions to start with:

- Keep a journal
- Simplify your life
- Eliminate unfulfilling parts of your life
- Find a healthy balance between work and play
- Don't isolate yourself
- Laugh
- Stop procrastinating
- Exercise
- Manage sleep better

When it seems like an emotional stressor may be causing problems, I have people keep a journal for thirty days. It can turn into a gratitude journal, or just a journal of what's bugging them, what's on their mind that day, or what they wake up thinking about in the middle of the night.

I also ask patients to consider simplifying their lives. Busyness seems to be a badge of honor in our society.

If you listen to people's conversations, you'll hear, "How are you, Martha?"

And Martha says, "Oh, I'm busy!"

To which the other person will often respond, "Oh, I'm busy too!"

I often ask patients if there are any tasks or obligations they can eliminate from their lives. We all need to start eliminating things that just keep us busy and that don't make us feel fulfilled. We need to learn to say no. We need to learn to find a healthy balance in our lives between play, work, and relaxation.

You especially need to *avoid isolation* when your stress is high. A lot of people will isolate themselves when they're really stressed, and that's when you most need to connect with friends and family, and with groups that give you emotional support.

Ways to connect with others include:

- Joining a civic group
- Going to church
- Taking a dance class
- Joining a choir
- Learning to play pickleball

You need to learn to *laugh often*. Start having fun, playing, and laughing! Most adults don't play. They don't even remember how to play. They don't laugh often, and life becomes so serious. Laughing and playing are so important for adults.

Try these activities to bring more laughter into your life:

- Attend a *Learn to Paint* party with friends
- Do a pottery project with friends or family
- Ride a zip line
- Jump out of an airplane

I advise you to *stop procrastinating*, because procrastination increases your stress level. You know you need to pay that bill, yet you procrastinate doing that. When you are late, you get a late fee, and it adds to your stress. So, stop procrastinating.

How can you stop procrastinating?

Plan three tasks to complete each day, no more, no less. Make it your goal to accomplish just those. After only a few days, you will feel a sense of accomplishment.

You also need to learn how to *exercise regularly* and you need to learn how to *sleep properly*. We'll talk about those two things next.

One more note: People who are suffering from stress need to go get their adrenals checked — as well as their blood sugar and their thyroid — by a practitioner who does an in-depth, deep dive. Primary care practitioners do not typically order the adrenal test; insurances usually don't cover it.

To get tested thoroughly, generally you need to find a good functional medicine practitioner who can do the testing and figure out what's going on with you. They can also provide you with information on nutraceuticals — medicines derived from food sources — botanicals, and lots of other things that functional practitioners learn in their course of training that can help people get better. I think the most important thing is to find a skilled practitioner who can restore your health in a functional manner.

EXERCISE — THE RIGHT AMOUNT OF THE RIGHT KIND FOR YOU

I was in my forties when I went through early menopause, and I started gaining weight. I went to my doctor, and a bunch of specialists. I went around looking for an answer to my weight issue.

All of them said, "Eat less, move more, and your weight will be just fine."

None of them thoroughly checked my thyroid, my cortisol levels, or my blood sugar. They just assumed I was eating too much and not moving enough. I then became determined to move more. I started race-walking, and I practiced hard. I became third in the nation for race walking — but I didn't lose any weight. I was very fit, but I didn't lose any weight. Then I decided I'd run marathons. I went to Honolulu, and I trained and completed a marathon. During that whole period — about seven months of extreme physical exertion and training — I lost maybe three pounds.

After I finished the marathon, my body was worn out. I had injuries, including chronic ingrown toenails, one of which I lost completely. Training for and running the marathon was extremely stressful for me and for my body, and I still hadn't lost the weight.

I think, like me, a lot of people take advice from a physician who's not really an expert in exercise. They try to follow the advice, and then they get discouraged that they aren't losing weight. That's one reason why I wanted to talk about exercise in this book. I've gone this route myself. I went after results, but followed the wrong path, so I understand how this can happen. But there is another way — a way that works — and I want to share it with you.

The Sitting of Today Is the Smoking of Twenty Years Ago

Twenty years ago, smoking was one of the highest risk factors for cardiovascular issues and diabetes. Today, people who are sedentary far outnumber smokers, and this sedentary lifestyle carries its own risks. Our society is a society of sitters; you sit in front of the TV, you sit in front of the computer; you sit all the time. People rarely even stand for any length of time. We don't exercise enough, and this has become very damaging to our bodies.

Do you have to sit at a desk for your job?

Many of us do, but there are ways to sit *actively*. By active sitting, I mean sitting on an exercise ball while you're typing or while you're watching TV or devoting regular time to active desk exercises while you are sitting. You can stand at an elevated desk while you're on your computer at work; you can remain standing at meetings. These tactics can truly enhance your cardiovascular health, but few people do them.

In my company, we have standing meetings all the time. Everyone stands at these meetings — and I mean *all* the employees in my organization — I've gotten pretty strict about it. I have more than one hundred employees. I'm the oldest of all of them, and I figure if I can stand for an hour at a meeting, the rest of them can, too. At these meetings, I let them know that we're not going to sit; we're going to stand—and at some point during the meeting, we will jump up and execute a *nitric oxide burst*. I'll talk about how to do that in a minute.

Sitting for long periods is damaging, and if you can create ways of getting up and moving—whether you get up and walk every half hour, do some desk exercises, do some pushups at your desk, move your arms, take a walk around the office complex—you can help reduce your risk of cardiovascular disease.

The high amount of sedentary client action is an independent risk factor for chronic disease, independent from the other amount of physical activity you do on a daily basis.

People often think that if they sit all day at their desk, but go to the gym afterwards and exercise, this will reduce their risk. That's not so. They need to incorporate movement into their day in addition to the trip to the gym after work. You can't erase sitting all day with an exercise burst in the evening. You've got to do it all day long.

High-Intensity Interval Training and Nitric Oxide Bursts

Most of the patients whom I treat do not come in already having a good exercise program. They may go out and walk the dog once a day. That's fine. That's great. That's good for their mental health, that's good for their heart, that's good for their body, but it's not going to get them the goals that they want. To truly improve your health and body condition, you need to adopt a good exercise program. It will help control your blood sugar levels, help you sleep well, improve your cardiovascular fitness, and will help you maintain good emotional health as well.

Be careful when you start a new training routine: a lot of people who push themselves with high-intensity aerobic training end up with injuries, especially if they're not in top-notch shape. If you overtrain, you will end up injuring yourself. If you train incorrectly, you can also injure yourself.

I highly recommend to my patients nitric oxide bursts—sometimes called *nitric oxide dump exercises*—and high-intensity interval training.

Nitric oxide bursts are simple and they don't take much time at all. In three-minute periods, two to three times a day, these exercises are designed to help your cardiovascular system relax. They also increase your *brain-derived neurotropic factor,* or BDNF, which acts like brain fertilizer, helping your neurons to grow.

There are videos on nitric oxide bursts that you can find on the internet. Dr. Joseph Mercola has a good YouTube video on nitric oxide bursts.

Here is the basic structure:

- Twenty squats — partial or full

- Twenty arm exercises, like you're doing a jumping jack but just using your arms

- Twenty overhead pushups without a weight

- You can add this exercise: Put your arms straight out in front of you, and move them up and down as fast as you can

- You can also add weights as you progress

A burst ends up being about three minutes of exercise, and it's an excellent exercise for sedentary people to do. Anybody who can get up out of a chair can do a squat, and whether it's a partial squat or a full-out squat, it's really good for the muscles. These exercises are a good thing to do in the office, first thing at the morning, at your lunch break, and before you leave. Nitric oxide bursts are an effective way to exercise. You should also include other forms of exercise in your plan, but nitric oxide bursts are a simple way to get started.

High-intensity interval training—or HIIT, as we call it—is different than what most people think. Most people think that if they get on the elliptical and go like crazy for an hour, that's high-intensity interval training. It's not. That is full-out aerobic training, which is not actually effective for weight loss, and is not as good for you as high-intensity interval training.

We start all of the patients who come through our clinic with high-intensity interval training, consisting of:

1. A four-minute warm-up, walking or standing in place—marching in place, riding on the bike at a gentle level—just to warm up your muscles

2. A thirty second push—if you're on the bike or the treadmill, speed up and go as fast as you can go. When your tongue is hanging out, that's when it's fast as you can go. Then you back off for four minutes.

3. Then you repeat the process.

Choose any interval training you want. You can run up and down stairs for thirty seconds. You can do squats with overhead pushups with weights. You can run back and forth as if you're playing tag, running from one side of the room to the other and touching the floor. Select exercises like these. Do four intervals of them. Overall, it takes about twenty minutes, after which you should always do a wind-down.

High-intensity interval training actually increases your fat burn for two hours. No other exercise increases your fat burn like high-intensity interval training, so I highly recommend it to patients. It doesn't take a massive amount of time. You don't have to join a gym. You can march in place if you want or run in place. You can go outside on the street and walk for four minutes, and then jog for thirty seconds. There are all kinds of ways of getting this exercise without a lot of expense and time.

Walking versus Running

I think all-out running is highly stressful. It is very hard on the body. Women who are marathon runners or long-distance runners often don't have periods. Commonly, there are a lot of injuries. Consider the Olympic long-distance runner; they don't have a lot of muscle mass on them, compared with a sprinter. A sprinter has a lot of muscle mass. In long-distance running, you don't develop muscle, and muscle is what is needed to burn calories.

Developing muscle has several benefits; for example, muscle mass:

- Helps us maintain physical fitness
- Helps to manage blood sugar, which is critical to avoid diabetes
- Is needed to keep body weight and body mass lower
- Gives us stability and balance

As we get older, we especially need that muscle mass to give us stability so that we don't tend to stumble and fall. There are a lot of reasons I believe — and there is a lot of research that supports my belief — that long-distance running is not the healthiest thing to do, in general. However, sometimes people will do the jog-run; they walk a little bit, then they jog a little bit. That's okay, because you're giving yourself a rest in between. If you want to do some long-distance running, you should walk in between. Walk for a few minutes, then run for a few minutes. It gives your body a break.

Jeff Galloway has written *The Run-Walk-Run Method* (Meyer & Meyer Sport, 2016) for people who like to run but have injuries that get in the way. The Galloway method eliminates injuries if followed properly. Jeff goes around the country teaching people how to walk and run to avoid injuries in long-distance running.

Finding a trainer who understands the latest research in exercise is important. If you need that level of expertise, hire a trainer. I had a trainer for years, until she went to nursing school, and I have since resorted to YouTube and DVD training tools that work well for my busy schedule. There are YouTube videos and online programs on high-intensity interval training that will take you from beginner to intermediate to advanced. You can get all kinds of information to help you on your journey to health.

SLEEPING ENOUGH AND SLEEPING WELL

Being a person who has suffered with insomnia, I know how important sleep is. Sleep management has always been an important part of treating patients in my practice, because if people don't sleep, they don't get better. That applies to both emotional and physical problems. One part of my practice is functional psychiatry, and I have found that the majority of those patients have trouble with sleep. I also work with a lot of menopausal women, or post-menopausal women. Menopause disrupts women's hormones, as well as their sleep.

I was an insomniac for years and years. I was taking prescription medications for sleep until I finally realized I couldn't go on long-term that way. I actually developed my own sleep formula and had it compounded. I made it available because I feel that most people don't have enough knowledge to create their own sleep formulas, so they end up messing with all kinds of different things, and often don't find a solution. I developed a compound that really works for me. *New Sleep* is my sleep formula and it can be found on my *Wellness Institute of Montana* website.

The Physiological Effects of Sleep

When you get high-quality sleep:

- Your body rebuilds cells.
- Your metabolism is boosted, which increases energy.
- Your immune system function is improved.
- Brain function is improved.
- Toxins that have built up are cleared.
- Lymph channels open up.
- Cerebral spinal fluid is increased.

A major function of sleep is to detoxify the brain. Sleep may be a way of clearing the brain of all the toxins that have accumulated from metabolism during the day. While you're awake, toxic substances, like free radicals, accumulate in the brain, and you have to get rid of them. You have to have a way of clearing the brain, and it happens in sleep.

Sleep is so important that if you go for a prolonged period without sleep, you can become dissociated from reality, and come into a state of psychosis. I treat a lot of patients for bipolar disorder. If they don't sleep for a couple of days, they can exhibit psychosis related to sleep deprivation.

Amyloids — protein fragments that are associated with dementia and Alzheimer's disease, which we will talk about in a later chapter — are cleared during sleep.

Memorization — the consolidation of memory — occurs with sleep. Your memories are stored for retrieval at this time. If you don't get good sleep, therefore, your ability to store memories for retrieval may be compromised. If you're wondering why you have so much difficulty memorizing things, it may be because you're not consolidating your thoughts at night while you're sleeping.

Sleep is critical, but its importance is often unappreciated. In our society, when we are extra busy, one of the first things that we sacrifice is sleep.

You start to say things like: *Oh, I'll get up at 3:00 in the morning and finish that, or, I'll just stay up late and finish that project.*

We give up sleep so easily, when we should really be guarding sleep ferociously.

In addition to the physiological health benefits of sleep, your willpower increases when you have good quality sleep. If you are reading this book, you are probably interested in getting healthier, and many of you may be trying to lose weight. Everything that has to do with health has to do with willpower. When sleep quality goes down, willpower goes down, so your chances of eating the pizza, the fries, the donuts, the sugar, and the ice cream all go up. Sleep is critical for the willpower that it takes to start and maintain an exercise program, buy and eat the correct foods, and do the right things for your body.

Sleep Hygiene

I give my patients a sleep hygiene sheet when they come in to see me, and I have done this for years.

What is on the list?

The first item on the list is to get a high coil count mattress. It will keep your neck and spine aligned. Get a good pillow. Consider whether you sleep on your side, your back, or your stomach because there are different pillows for all types of sleeping. Invest in natural fiber—like cotton or linen—sheets that don't have plastic or any preservatives in them, so your bedding is less toxic. These natural-fiber fabrics will actually help control your temperature better at night.

Cut out all nicotine, including smokeless tobacco. It is a stronger stimulant than caffeine. You should cut out caffeine as well; you shouldn't drink caffeine past noon. Make sure your thermostat in your bedroom is between 65°F and 67 °F. People generally sleep better when it's a little cooler.

Cover up the electric lights in your bedroom. One of my friends, when he travels, takes along a roll of duct tape, and he covers up the clocks and any of those annoying lights that are in the room. The darker you can make the room, the better you will sleep.

Don't use electronic computers, laptops, TVs, and so on, beyond an hour before bedtime. This advice is about avoiding the lights on these screens, so it is okay to listen to music or to a story. If you have to use an electronic screen in the evening, you can wear blue spectrum blocking glasses for a couple of hours before bedtime, and that will help.

Create a pre-sleep routine of a hot bath or a warm Jacuzzi, or something similar that is relaxing. Soothe your soul with music, meditation, yoga, or light reading. Write down your worries; get them out of your head. Sometimes, just writing down what's on your mind helps. Keep a list by your bed; if you wake up with a worry on your mind, write it down, and go back to sleep.

Set regular hours of sleep that coincide with your natural circadian rhythm, rising and resting when possible with the rhythm of the sun. Avoid sleeping in on weekends. You should keep a regular circadian rhythm. I know this is one of the hardest things for shift workers to do; they really struggle with their sleep.

Use your bedroom and bed only for sleep and sex. Only these two activities should happen in the bedroom. If you lie awake more than twenty minutes, get up, leave the bedroom, and go read something boring, then go back to bed. Don't stay in the bed more than twenty minutes if you're awake.

It's critical that you determine whether you have sleep apnea. When you're having difficulty sleeping, take a test to see if you have sleep apnea. You can conduct an overnight test in your home, often free of charge, from an oxygen company. If you do have sleep apnea, you'll have to fix that before you're ever going to get adequate or regenerative sleep.

Nutraceutical Approaches

Many nutraceuticals and botanicals can improve sleep.

Nutraceuticals are medicines derived from food sources. Pharmaceuticals are developed in labs and frequently use components that are far from food and plant sources.

If you go to a primary care doctor, it is likely you will get a prescription for Ambien or Lunesta. There are lots of prescription drugs for sleep, but all of them have side effects. Sometimes side effects can include sleep behaviors like night walking, eating during the middle of the night, or going outside and driving during the middle of your sleep. In these cases, prescription medications may not be the safest way to go.

After you incorporate all of the sleep hygiene recommendations in the last section, you may want to work with a functional medicine practitioner to try some nutraceuticals.

Some that may help with sleep are listed below:

- Melatonin
- Progesterone
- Gaba
- Valerian
- Magnesium
- L-theanine
- Tart cherry juice
- Passionflower

Some of the natural products may be more potent if you take them together, if you have a lot of trouble sleeping. *Melatonin* is an over-the-counter product that you can easily find, and I usually recommend one to three milligrams. Our body makes melatonin, but you might just need a little bit more. If you're a woman with sleep difficulties and your progesterone level is down, you can see if taking progesterone at night will help you. You would have to ask your primary care doctor or your functional medicine doctor about that.

Other choices are gaba (gamma-amino butyric acid), valerian, and magnesium. Magnesium is a wonderful sleep enhancer, and it also relaxes your muscles. If you're having restless leg system, which a lot of people have, a little magnesium can help with that. You can try l-theanine, tart cherry juice, or passionflower. There are many nutraceuticals available for you to try, and you may find that taking several in combination works better than just one or two. See your health professional for advice.

One non-nutraceutical approach that I tried for quite a while was using software that promotes *delta-wave sleep*. You can get some programs online—audio programs that are free. You put your earphones on and listen to the sounds and music as you go to sleep. Look for insomnia programs online that help with the delta-wave sleep. They really seem to work well if you can sleep with earphones in for at least an hour or two—if they fall out after the first hour, that's okay. These programs may help put you to sleep without having to take any sleep medication.

CHAPTER THREE

Different Food Plans

PALEO

In general, there is a lot of confusion about diets. When I struggled with weight gain in my late forties and early fifties, I tried every diet I could, including Weight Watchers, South Beach, and Atkins. I'd hear about a diet, read about it, and I'd try it.

I think the confusion about diets has largely been initiated by the food industry, because our culture dishes out bad choices every day. There is confusion from the food industry, the diet industry, pharmaceuticals, and books. They keep people confused because you can sell a confused person anything, and they will try it. That's what I did.

Most people don't start looking for a diet until they become overweight. In the functional medicine world, the time to start looking for a lifestyle food plan is before you get sick, before you get obese.

But no matter when you start thinking about changing your diet, keep in mind that the foods you eat reflect the way you live. Food is an important part of lifestyle. Food also has the ability to turn on and turn off DNA, so it is very powerful.

Your new diet must be specific to the condition that you are treating, and for your unique needs — both your nutritional needs and your lifestyle needs. We have to find the diet that works for you and your family. Since the recipient of the diet or the lifestyle food plan is going to be eating or sharing it with their family, we always look at the whole family. We're treating the patients and their families before we ever pick out a food plan.

One other note: many packaged foods are truly manufactured to cause addiction in people. There are people employed in the food industry whose job it is to make foods addictive, so that we just can't get enough of it. With that said, I'd like to say that figuring out how to change the nutritional plan you're on, or should be on, is like flying a plane.

If I gave you a manual on piloting a plane and you read it, would you then go jump in the plane and try to fly it?

Most people wouldn't. It's the same way with nutrition. Once you find what your body needs, based on your condition, then you will need help learning how to shop and how to find the foods that work. You will need recipes; you will need to learn how to prepare the foods. There's a whole skill set on how to learn to feed yourself in a healthy way. Even though you've been feeding yourself for years, this will be a learning experience.

What Is the Paleo Diet?

Chris Kresser is a well-known practitioner of integrative and functional medicine, and he has written and studied a lot about the Paleo diet. I recommend his book, *The Paleo Cure* (Little and Brown, 2014). He started down the road of the Paleo diet because he, himself, was very sick. Paleo diets in general follow the lifestyle of the hunter-gatherer forebearers. Simply put, Paleo is based on what the members of these hunter-gatherer tribes all over the world ate. When berries were in season, they ate berries. When they killed a buffalo, they ate the buffalo, and all of its parts.

Who Can Benefit from a Paleo Diet?

I think Paleo is a good starting point for most people, just for general health. If they don't know particularly what's wrong with them, it's a safe place to start. Anyone can benefit from a version of the basic Paleo diet. You can do a Paleo for autoimmune support, or other specific problems, a Paleo for reboot, or a Paleo for weight loss. The basic concept of the Paleo diet is there are foods that you eat liberally, there are foods that you eat in moderation, and then there are foods that you avoid completely.

Paleo Diet Foods to Eat Liberally

Meat, poultry, and wild game are in this category. Chicken, duck, goat, anything that's organic and free-range is acceptable. You want to minimize toxins, so you don't want to go to the grocery store and buy beef that's been raised in a confined agricultural factory farm. It's best to buy local. Some factory farms claim their animals are grass-fed, but the animals may not be reliably contained. You have to be really careful where you source all of your foods. Buy local whenever you can.

Organ meats are especially important—liver, for example—because they're very nutrient-dense in vitamins, iron, and essential amino acids. Bone broth is a wonderful food to heal your gut. It's rich in glycine and amino acids that you need for your gut lining. Homemade bone broth is great, but sometimes you can buy good homemade bone broth soup in the grocery store.

You should eat three six-ounce servings of fish per week to get enough omega-3s, with a proper EPA-

DHA ratio. Small fish — and wild fish, if possible — are recommended. Eggs should be free-range and organic if possible, and yes, yolks are allowed. There's no problem with yolks; they are full of nutrition.

When it comes to vegetables, there's a bountiful list. Starchy plants — such as sweet potatoes, tapioca, yuccas, plantains, and breadfruits — are allowed on the Paleo diet but must be eaten in moderation. You can eat the non-starchy vegetables, either cooked or raw. That includes a lot of the green tops of plants. With a few exceptions, if it's green, you can eat it. The same for red, like beets and grapes. Mushrooms are also included in this group.

You can eat as many fermented vegetables and fruits as you want on a Paleo diet. Some examples are lacto-fermented sauerkraut, kimchi, kvass, and coconut kefir. They're loaded with good bacteria that help your gut health.

The fats allowed in the Paleo diet are coconut oil, ghee, palm kernel oil, macadamia oil, lard, and olive oil, preferably extra virgin olive oil. Other fat-rich items that are allowed are olives, avocados, and coconuts.

Also use sea salt and spices. You can use raw, unfiltered apple cider vinegar — the kind with the *mother* intact. It's especially useful in salad dressings.

Paleo Foods to Eat in Moderation

Processed meat and whole fruits should be consumed in moderation. Depending on your blood sugar balance, you can eat two to three servings of fruit a day, but if you have blood sugar problems, fruit will contribute to these problems. Generally, if you're trying to lose weight, you would cut back to one serving of berries a day. Nuts and seeds are very nutrient-dense, but they're also very good for you. The best nuts are almonds and Brazil nuts, cashews, hazelnuts, macadamias, walnuts, pine nuts, and pecans.

There are a few vegetables, including green beans, sugar peas, and snap peas, which are technically in the greens, but are limited in the Paleo diet. Coffee and tea should be limited to one or two cups per day.

Paleo Foods to Avoid Completely

If you are aiming to have a good, healthy lifestyle, you will find there will be some foods you will be advised to avoid. In a Paleo diet, you want to avoid all processed, refined foods that come in boxes or packages, or have preservatives. You want to avoid dairy, especially if you have a sensitivity to dairy. You will also avoid most grains, especially wheat, rye, and oats—unless they're processed in a gluten-free factory. Rice and quinoa are fine. Avoid legumes, sweeteners, industrial or factory meats, vegetable oil, chocolate—unless it's seventy percent cocoa or more—all sodas—including diet sodas or fruit-sweetened sodas—fruit juice, and alcohol.

In restaurant kitchens, industrial meats and vegetable oils are often used for cooking. These foods are hard on your system, so you have to be very proactive in restaurants—letting your server know what you want your vegetables sautéed in, and how you want your food cooked.

You shouldn't eat processed sauces and seasonings because they usually include sugar, corn gluten, or other items on the avoidance list.

FOOD PLANS FROM THE INSTITUTE OF FUNCTIONAL MEDICINE

As a practitioner, I have gone through the Institute of Functional Medicine (IFM) training course. It's approximately a three-year training course focused on techniques in functional medicine: how to look at root causes and how to treat them. Nutrition plays a big role in functional medicine, as we've already discussed.

Dietary needs are different for each patient, and for every chronic health condition, there is a nutritious food plan that would benefit the patient. Once you have identified a chronic condition, by working with your functional medicine practitioner and getting the proper labs and tests done, then your functional practitioner will know which kind of plan you need to eat for life, or until your condition improves.

The IFM curriculum includes a great deal of nutrition education that I have found exceptionally valuable. It has developed several specialized diets, or main lifestyle food plans, and they're all based on research. The IFM makes their references available to practitioners, so we can read up on all of the diets. They're well-researched plans, and often have elements that are contrary to commonly found diet advice—like the Standard American Diet (SAD), the American food plan, My Plate, or the food pyramid.

I really like the IFM diets because I know they are based on current research, while other diet plans may not be well researched, or may not be based on up-to-date information. These diet plans are made available to practitioners in the IFM training courses. I'll give a brief description of some of them below. Ask your medical practitioner about the IFM diet plan that best fits your particular health needs.

The IFM Core Plan

IFM has a basic, core plan, in addition to their specialized plans. It's a great starting point for someone who doesn't have any significant health problems, for someone who just wants to start eating right.

Here are the basic characteristics of the IFM Core Plan:

- The plan consists of whole foods and promotes clean, organic types of eating.

- There's *phytonutrient diversity,* meaning there's a diversity of color in the vegetables of this food plan. Each different color has a different set of nutrients that it brings into your body, making this diversity beneficial.

- It has adequate, quality protein in it, and a healthy quantity of good-quality fats.

- It's high in fiber and low in sugar.

- Elimination of most processed foods is encouraged.

- In the core diet, there's no calorie restriction. There's no emphasis on reducing carbs, fats, or fasting.

The IFM Core Plan is an easy-to-follow diet. Dairy-free, gluten-free, and grain-free versions are optional. I would put anyone on this diet as a foundational eating plan. The core food plan is a good one for eating right. Paleo is a good foundational eating plan as well.

The Elimination Diet

As I mentioned earlier, any patient who comes into my practice is put on an elimination diet because, often, if you can eliminate a common food sensitivity, the person's condition improves. Instead of starting with a bunch of expensive testing, I'll put them on the elimination diet while I'm waiting for some of their basic blood labs and stool specimens to come back.

In the elimination diet, there is generally no calorie restriction. It is dairy-free and gluten-free, with an option of grain-free. Besides helping to identify food triggers, this diet promotes body awareness of food. People on the elimination diet will notice right away if they start sleeping better, or if their arthritic pain decreases. We eliminate sugar in the elimination diet, because once you do that, you reduce inflammation, you support the gut, you promote the nutrients that are needed to heal the gut, and you reduce the toxic burden in the body.

The Cardio-Metabolic Diet

I own and operate a mental health center where obesity is a big problem largely due to the side effects of psychotropic medications. I have introduced the *cardio-metabolic diet* into the mental health center as well as into the group homes and the Alzheimer's unit because so many of those folks have diabetes or cardiovascular problems. The cardio diet is for people with cardiovascular problems, obesity, diabetes, and related conditions.

The cardio-metabolic diet has these characteristics:

- It's targeted with respect to calories, so there is a calorie restriction. I figure out what the restrictions should be, based on each patient's lean body mass.

- It has a balanced quality of fats.

- It's high in fiber and low in simple sugars.

- It's got a very low-glycemic impact, so it doesn't affect blood sugar much.

- Elimination of processed foods is optional but encouraged.

- It is kind of a modified Mediterranean diet, which a lot of people like, especially if they like fish.

- The phytonutrients in the diet are specifically chosen to help heal a cardiovascular metabolic problem.

This diet can help balance blood sugar, support cardiovascular health, and manage weight. People with cardio-metabolic problems, such as heart, blood pressure, obesity, and diabetes would especially benefit from the cardio-metabolic diet.

The Renew Food Plan

The renew food plan eliminates all processed and refined foods and includes a high level of phytonutrient diversity. This kind of food plan helps to identify and reduce food triggers. It's dairy-free, gluten-free, grain-free, and sugar-free. It's useful for people who have inflammation, especially those who have some type of gut problem—whether it's IBS, *gastroesophageal reflux disease* (GERD), or leaky gut—and it helps reduce cravings and food addiction. It encourages the healthy elimination of toxins, and it supports sugar detoxification. The renew plan is what I would use for someone who clearly has a sugar addiction or a bread addiction. We see many people who have these addictions.

The Mito Food Plan

The *mito* in this IFM food plan is short for *mitochondria*. Every cell in our body has energy structures that are called mitochondria. They are what create molecules of *adenosine tri-phosphate* (ATP), which is where energy is stored for life processes. When mitochondria don't work properly, this can cause many physiological issues, including neurodegenerative problems.

The mitochondrial diet is relatively strict. It has some *ketogenic* options, which we'll discuss in more detail in the next section.

This diet has reduced carbs and a higher fat—good fat—content than a normal diet would have, and there is intermittent fasting and calorie restriction involved. It is usually recommended that, after dinnertime, you don't eat again for twelve to sixteen hours. A lot of people fast for sixteen hours, and then have an eight-hour window to eat. It is very low in grains, and gluten is not included in this plan whatsoever, because gluten can trigger a lot of mitochondrial inflammation.

The mito food plan is designed to reduce inflammation. People think inflammation is only in the joints, but any tissue can be affected by it. You can have inflammation in your brain, and brain inflammation is a factor associated with Alzheimer's. Besides assisting with inflammation issues, the mito plan has a very low-glycemic impact, so it helps to balance your blood sugar. It provides targeted antioxidants. Because it has good quality dietary fats, it is good for energy. Of all the diets, the mito diet is the most restrictive diet, and it is especially good for anyone who has a neurodegenerative disorder, or Alzheimer's.

THE KETOGENIC DIET

Most people have a loved one who has dementia or know someone in their family who has died from dementia. Most Americans perceive dementia as a terminal illness. The good news is—*it is not*. With lifestyle changes, including the ketogenic diet that we will discuss here, you may be able to reduce your risk substantially.

In this section, I want to make sure that you understand what *ketosis* is, and what a ketogenic diet is, compared with what you may have heard.

What Is a Ketogenic Diet?

When you hear the word *ketogenic,* you may think of diabetics and ketoacidosis.

In a ketogenic state, your body and brain are using ketones for energy instead of the easier-to-use glucose. Ketones are pulled from the fat stored in your body.

Our bodies have a unique ability to use carbs, fats, and proteins for energy. Our bodies prefer carbs. It's much easier to take a carb, turn it into glucose, take the glucose and transport it into the cell, where the cell can happily use the glucose. The extra glucose that is not used is then stored as fat. Insulin stores a lot of glucose as fat, but our brains are very sensitive to glucose. They don't like glucose.

With the ketogenic diet, which is very low in carbs, we have to find a different source of energy. If you're on a really low-carb diet, the body's preference is fat; the body can become a fat-burning machine. We have to get into ketosis to make our bodies start desiring ketones over carbohydrates. Body fat is converted to ketones, which are a sustainable and stable energy source. By limiting carb intake, the body will remain in ketosis, which not only helps you lose weight, but also helps your brain function more efficiently. The ketogenic diet is important for burning fat, which helps address problems for diabetics, patients with cardiovascular disease, and all the obese people in the world. More importantly, the ketogenic food plan is the diet—a very strict one—that you need for the prevention and reversal of Alzheimer's.

The ketogenic diet has been around for a long time. It started in the early 1940s, when it was used for kids with epileptic seizures. It's still very popular and very effective for people with seizures. There's a lot of good information out on the ketogenic diet. The ketogenic diet is not the same as the Atkins diet, which came out in 1972. The Atkins diet is heavy on proteins, while the ketogenic diet is heavier on fats and less on proteins because proteins can be converted into a form of glucose and used as energy.

The ketogenic diet is very low in carbs, very high in fat, and moderate in proteins.

In the Standard American Diet, the diet consists of about 30 percent fats, 20 percent protein, and 50 percent carbs. In a ketogenic diet, we're looking at approximately 70 percent fats, 10 percent carbohydrates, and 20 percent protein—note that the amount of protein recommended really depends on your lean body mass.

You should not take on this diet by yourself. Make sure you have a practitioner to guide you, so you can take in the proper percentage of macronutrients—fats, carbs, and proteins—for your body size and goals.

A ketogenic diet pyramid is an inverse pyramid, really, of what the Standard American Diet is.

The base of the pyramid is divided in two.

On one side are:

- Healthy oils and fats: butter, olive oil, coconut oil, MCT (medium chain triglycerides) oil
- Avocados
- Nuts

The diet allows a liberal use of the oils in cooking, on your salads, and all day long, even in your smoothies.

On the other side of the pyramid base are:

- Fatty fish
- Meats
- Organ meats
- Eggs, including the yolk

In the middle of the pyramid, you have:

- Green vegetables
- Nonstarchy vegetables, such as kale, cucumbers, asparagus, and zucchini

As you move up, you get into:

- Nightshades, such as peppers and tomatoes

- Vegetables that are low in carbs, such as broccoli, and onions

Then above that, there is:

Raw, full-fat dairy

At the very top, there are:

- Nuts
- Seeds
- Berries

There is no processed, refined food on this pyramid. Neither are there grains. You're not going to be eating bread, gluten-free or otherwise. It's a pretty strict diet, but it's also a clean and simple diet.

Who Would Benefit from a Ketogenic Diet?

I recently went to a conference where I was trained in Dr. Dale Bredesen's *ReCODE Protocol,* a program to help people avoid or reverse Alzheimer's. The ketogenic diet pays a crucial role in how well patients do with respect to reversing or preventing Alzheimer's. Dr. Bredesen recommends that all people, at age forty-five, get a checkup from a trained practitioner who knows about preventing and reversing dementia or cognitive decline, and start there. If genetic testing shows they have the ApoE-4 gene, which indicates a possible predisposition to Alzheimer's, they need to start on the ketogenic diet when they're forty-five. You can get tested for the ApoE-4 gene, and then go see the practitioner trained in ReCODE protocol and they'll set up a program.

The ketogenic diet is also useful with all kinds of neurological conditions, like Parkinson's and MS, and for those with type 2 diabetes. That, to me, is quite amazing because in the diabetic nutrition world, the focus is often on grains and bread exchanges. However, for someone with diabetes who practices a ketogenic diet, their blood sugars may be stabilized by this kind of food plan, which includes no grains.

The ketogenic food plan can also be helpful in reducing your high blood pressure and your cholesterol, and it's useful for inflammation because it omits many of the inflammatory foods. In addition, even though you're eating 70 percent fats, it actually lowers your triglycerides, which are really a byproduct of sugar in your diet, and increases your HDL—your good cholesterol. It's certainly a win-win for a lot of folks with lots of different conditions.

Sample Foods from a Ketogenic Diet

Here is a typical day on a ketogenic diet:

You might start the day with a baked spinach-cheese omelet, with a half-cup of dairy. You would have a snack of a couple almonds in the middle of the morning.

For lunch, you could have a quick salmon or tuna salad, mixed greens, and pepper strips, with MCT oil or a vinaigrette. MCT is a good oil for the ketogenic diet because very little is stored as fat and it is used for energy very quickly.

Then you would have another snack in the afternoon: maybe two tablespoons of pistachio nuts, or some seaweed flake squares.

Then for dinner, you might have smoked brisket, roasted vegetables, and mushrooms and bell peppers sautéed with arugula. The roasted vegetables and sautéed vegetables you would cook in olive oil or coconut oil.

As you can see, the diet is really heavy on vegetables and fat.

That would be a typical day on a ketogenic diet, without intermittent fasting. Intermittent fasting is recommended if you have Alzheimer's or cognitive decline.

Some people say: *I don't know how I can possibly get all of those phytonutrients in my day! We're busy people! How do you eat like that?*

There's a lot of planning required. You have to plan your menu for the week, and you have to make the time to buy your vegetables and produce that you need.

You might think: *I don't have time to make an omelet in the morning. I have kids to get off to school. I need to get to work.*

Smoothies

Smoothies are a simple way to deliver a good dose of vitamins, minerals, and essential nutrients. You can learn to make them for quick breakfasts that give great nutrition. Experiment with different foods to see which ingredients you like best. Vegetables and fruits can be washed and cut up ahead, so prep time in the morning shouldn't take very long.

A good smoothie should start with four to six ounces of a base liquid. Base liquids can be coconut milk, almond milk, or two to four ounces of unsweetened juice.

I generally put a half-cup of berries in mine. You can use one to two cups of whole vegetables. Not all vegetables taste good in a smoothie—the ones that are probably best are cucumbers, spinach leaves, or zucchini. They are pretty neutral.

Then you can add two tablespoons of protein—ten to twenty grams of protein. You can use yogurt or kefir as the protein source. You can also add nut butters or commercial protein powders. However, you have to be very careful about commercial protein powders because some of them are full of sugar or preservatives. Read the labels carefully.

Adding avocado, a good source of fat, will make the smoothie creamier.

Add some ground flaxseed for some good omega-3s. Then you're set to go. Whip it up with some ice cubes, and you've got a pretty nutritious breakfast.

In summary, a good basic recipe for smoothies is:

- 4–6 ounces base liquid: nut milks or unsweetened fruit juice

- ½ cup berries or fruit: green apples, blueberries, banana

- 1–2 cups fresh vegetables: cucumber, zucchini, kale, or spinach

- 10–20 grams (2 tablespoons) protein: whey or hemp powder, yogurt, or nut butters

- Omega-3s: a tablespoon of flaxseed, fish oil, or a handful of soaked nuts

- Ice, if desired

One final benefit to smoothies: If you are taking a lot of nutritional products, a lot of people will buy the liquid form and pour the liquid into their smoothies or open some of the capsules and dump them into the smoothies. This way they don't have to swallow as many capsules.

For most of these diets, or if you have a chronic health condition, you really need to find a functional practitioner who knows how to manage your condition and understands what lifestyle food plan you should be on.

When you're on the ketogenic diet, you will need to test your urine or your blood. If a ketogenic person is in cognitive decline, you're going to want to do a finger stick with a meter to check your blood for sugar and ketones at the same time. If you're eating a proper percentage of fats, proteins, and carbs, your blood sugar should run in the lower range of normal, and you should be burning a lot of ketones. There are strips that test blood and urine for ketones and sugar. When you first start the diet, your practitioner will keep checking until they figure out where your levels should be.

CHAPTER FOUR

The Brain—Prevention and Reversal of Alzheimer's

THE TOP THREE CAUSES OF ALZHEIMER'S

Alzheimer's disease is an epidemic in the United States and all over the world. It is in the top five causes of death in the United States today. There are 5 million people in the U.S. who have active Alzheimer's disease, according the *2017 Alzheimer's Disease Facts and Figures*. It is projected that there will be 16 million by 2050. The unpaid caregiving cost is $230 billion—that's the cost of caregivers leaving from their jobs to stay home and take care of their loved ones. The medical costs in 2017 to our nation were $259 million, predicted to rise to 1.1 trillion by 2050.

My greatest concern about Alzheimer's, besides having personal experience with it, is that this one disease could bring Medicare and Medicaid to its knees in the next couple of generations. It needs our attention now.

The traditional approach for Alzheimer's begins when a patient consults their doctor about some memory loss.

That patient is likely to hear statements like these:

- *There's nothing that will prevent, reverse, or slow the process of Alzheimer's.*

- *Everyone knows someone who is a cancer survivor. No one knows an Alzheimer's survivor.*

- *You need to get your final plans and your will prepared. Quit driving and take care of end-of-life issues.*

I recently read a similar statement from a neuropsychologist to whom I had referred a patient. My patient had gotten a new diagnosis of Alzheimer's but no plan, no hope, nothing to help him through this disease.

To me, it's pretty amazing that the word is still not out to the public that this is a disease that is reversible and preventable. I think it's critical to get the word out that Alzheimer's is no longer a death sentence.

Alzheimer's is not a death sentence, but it *is* a sneaky reaper. I say it's a sneaky reaper because it is possible for a patient to have up to one decade of subjective cognitive impairment before diagnosis. During this period, the patient may notice they're forgetting people's names, faces, where they left their keys, or how to get to the store. This may be followed by a few years of mild cognitive impairment, where other people notice that the patient is forgetting. Then it comes to full-blown Alzheimer's, and the person begins to lose their ability to function and do their regular activities.

Most people in the United States are waiting for a drug to cure Alzheimer's. They don't realize that in Alzheimer's, there are at least forty things that go wrong in the brain. It's like a roof with forty holes in it. A drug may fill one or two holes, but then you still have thirty-eight holes in your roof.

What people don't realize is there are three main causes that trigger Alzheimer's:

1. Inflammation
2. Deficiencies in hormones and nutrition
3. Toxins

Inflammation

Inflammation is from infections. It could be a *stealth infection,* when you don't even know you have an infection. This happens in the gut due to an unregulated immune system; a lot of people have bacteria in the gut, or yeast, or other parasites. They don't even know they have them, but the body responds with inflammation. The diet can also be inflammatory. If you have a gluten sensitivity or a dairy sensitivity and you're eating those foods, this can cause inflammation in your body.

The only way to figure out if you're inflamed is having a health professional who takes a good medical history and orders the right lab tests. There are a lot of inflammatory markers that you can order on blood tests. It is possible to know of a patient's inflammation as soon as I get blood levels back from the lab. I begin by looking at inflammatory markers, and if there's an inflammatory marker, I then have to find the root cause of that inflammation.

Deficiencies

Most Americans eat the Standard American Diet. They may take a multivitamin, or they may take vitamin D because they have heard that it is good for you. Very few of the patients I treat come to me having adequate nutritional supplements, and if they are taking supplements, often they are picking them up off the shelf in a drugstore, and they don't know the potency or quality of the contents. They don't know if the bottle actually contains the product it claims to contain, and at what percentage — most of the time, the supplements are not pure.

The average diet is so insufficient today because our soils have become depleted; our farmlands no longer have the minerals in the soil that we need. So, between selecting a bad diet, eating foods that don't have the nutritional value that they used to have, and taking supplement products of questionable value, many people are suffering nutritional deficiencies.

There are also supplemental hormones to consider. A lot of people are taking statin drugs. Statin drugs affect cholesterol level, and cholesterol is a precursor to many hormones in your body. You need to have cholesterol for cell function. If a man consults me with some subjective symptoms of cognitive impairment, I will test his testosterone level to see what's going on. If a woman seeks my expertise, I check her estrogen, progesterone, and testosterone, to make sure that those hormones are adequate.

Another set of hormones are the thyroid hormones. You cannot have a healthy brain if you don't have a healthy thyroid, and you can't have a healthy thyroid if you have an inflamed gut.

You can see that everything works together. There is no one single cause of Alzheimer's. There are a lot of factors that work together to trigger problems in your body, and you have to go after all of them. You can't just pick one or two things; you need to address all of them.

Toxins

Toxins are everywhere. When you start talking about toxins to people, they start looking at you like you're kind of *out there*. Americans do not realize how full of toxins our environment is.

Several years ago, while I was getting functional medicine training, I went through a three-day toxin course — three days, just on toxins. In my training to become a registered nurse, I'd never heard about toxins. In my nurse practitioner training, they never talked about toxins.

When I began the functional medicine toxin course, I thought: *Okay, they're going a little overboard with toxins.*

But as I learned more, I regarded the topic more seriously, and it wasn't long before I was saying to myself: *Okay, I'm not drinking out of plastic bottles any more.*

I researched the cosmetics and hair products I was using. I considered the quality of air in my home. As we've already discussed, you can get several tests to check out the toxin levels in your home. Some of the most damaging toxins that affect your brain are from metal. Around your home, you can be exposed to toxins from metals such as mercury, lead, or a whole variety of metals present in paint, water, or other sources.

Investigate the toxins in your environment, especially those that may trigger your allergies, or impact conditions you may have. I have asthma, and I found out that there is chlorine in our city's water. Chlorine can contribute to asthma. You have to look at everything around you when you're looking for toxins.

Then, there are *biotoxins*. Biotoxins are dangerous. Mold is the biotoxin that people are most commonly affected by. If you live in a home that's old, has had roof leakage, if water has gotten into the insulation, the basement has gotten wet, or you've experienced any type of flood – even a toilet overflowing and going through the walls – these conditions can lead to mold exposure. Sometimes mold is obvious in a home, but sometimes it's not obvious. You can get an inexpensive mold-testing kit online, dust your house, and see if you have mold spores. If you do, you must get rid of them to get your brain healthier, or to avoid dementia.

With the top three causes of Alzheimer's, all three of them are reversible or preventable. To me, that's the good news. Alzheimer's is the bad news, but the good news is, you can treat it. The process that leads to Alzheimer's – the amyloid response in your brain – is protective, initially. It's there to help clean up debris and damaged cells. Amyloids in themselves are not bad, and the amyloid response is a natural process. One reason Alzheimer's comes when that process is out of balance is because we are bombarding our brains with so many bugs, toxins, and traumas that it can't keep up.

GENETIC TESTING

I want to ask, "How do you give yourself Alzheimer's?"

No one ever talks about it that way, but I want to open with that.

As I've discussed, there are approximately forty factors that influence the health of the brain, with new factors being researched. You give yourself Alzheimer's when you live your life in a way that keeps your brain supplied with as many of those forty factors as possible. You live your life this way, and then you don't identify that you have a genetic predisposition for Alzheimer's. That's the ApoE-4 gene, and I'll talk about that more in depth.

People are giving themselves Alzheimer's by continuing with the Standard American Diet, having little to no exercise, spending a lot of time sitting, lacking mental stimulation, and becoming very isolated as they become older, so they don't have social interaction. They don't go to a practitioner who identifies their deficiencies in vitamins and hormones. They ignore any inflammatory symptoms; they just live with them or take over-the-counter pain relief. They disregard toxins in their environment. If people continue this way, all of these items together are a setup for Alzheimer's.

The ApoE-4 Gene

We are all born with lots — and lots, and lots — of genes. More are identified through research every year. Genes contain predispositions. When we're talking about the ApoE-4 gene, it's important to understand that, even if you have zero copies of the gene, you still have a 9 percent lifetime risk of getting Alzheimer's because of lifestyle. All of the contributing factors I talked about in the last section — about how to give yourself Alzheimer's — also refer to the people with the 9 percent, the zero copies. Without the gene, you can still get it. If you have one copy of the ApoE-4 gene, you have a 30 percent lifetime risk of getting dementia. If you have two copies — referred to as *homozygous* for that gene — you have a 50–90 percent lifetime risk of getting dementia.

As you can see, it's critical to identify early what your genetic predisposition is, and to start treating it aggressively to prevent or reverse cognitive decline. The *23 and Me* genomics company offers a genetic test, which my husband and I recently took. This company not only offers ancestry DNA data; it will also will give you medical DNA data for an additional fee. If you find a practitioner like me, we will upload your data, get the raw data, and get a lot more information for you about your genes. Then we can sit down, share it with you, talk with you about your data, and counsel you on what you need to do with this information.

On a personal note about the ApoE-4 gene: I've always been interested in Alzheimer's. As a younger nursing administrator, I set up and operated three Alzheimer's units, and I currently own an Alzheimer's unit in one of my assisted living homes. I would much rather cure that disease than treat the end results of that disease.

Even more personally, I got married this year, and on my honeymoon, we got an email from *23 and Me*. My genes were clear; I had no ApoE-4 gene. My husband, my brand-new husband, had two. He's homozygous for ApoE-4, and he's seventy-two years old. I was already interested and had taken training in the reversal of Alzheimer's, but this new information has given me even more of a drive to help people avoid and prevent Alzheimer's. He and I together are trying to work a program— that I'll talk about in a little while—to reverse or to avoid any cognitive decline. He doesn't have any obvious symptoms at this time, and so our job is to work together to keep him that way. I'm living the life of the ApoE-4 caregiver already, so it's a pretty important topic for me.

Genetic Testing: How to Get It Done and What the Results Mean

All a person has to do is go online. There are several genetic testing sites, but the least expensive—and it gives good information—is *23 and Me*. You just go online and sign up for the program. The cost, with the genetic testing, is around $200 at the time of the writing of this book. You'll be asked lots of questions, because *23 and Me* is gathering data on participants' backgrounds and symptoms to help with research on different genes. You can get involved in their research, so it's kind of fun. It gives us in the scientific community a lot more information.

It's easy to do the *23 and Me* test. It takes a couple of weeks to get the results, and once you get the results, you have to find either a program online to upload the raw data to—for a fee—or you find a practitioner who has the knowledge to do that for you. Your primary care doctor will probably not know what all the genes and the genetic variables mean, nor within the span of what feels like ever-shortening primary-care visits will you get the time to go over your genetic testing. Look for a functional medicine practitioner instead, to help you review your genetic test results, and figure out a plan of attack if necessary. Anyone over age forty-five needs to get this done.

PREVENTION AND TREATMENT OF ALZHEIMER'S

Again, Alzheimer's is preventable, and it's reversible in the early stages. The more you know about your own personal risk, or your loved one's risk, the more you can do to prevent it. Another recommendation I make is for a *cognoscopy*—a workup to see what your risk is, how healthy you are, and how well you will go through aging.

Everybody at age forty-five should get a cognoscopy, which consists of a:

- Smell test

- Walking speed test

- Genetic test—making sure you have your ApoE-4 done

- Full set of labs: adrenal testing, lipid testing, full thyroid testing, metabolic markers, inflammatory markers, and tests for toxins when indicated

Some people may need an MRI with body metrics as well—if they have the ApoE-4 gene, or if they have subjective cognitive impairment symptoms.

How to Treat Inflammation, How to Treat Deficiencies, and Removal of Toxins

The entire ReCODE prevention program is directed at treating inflammation, deficiencies, and toxins.

First, you optimize the diet. The best diet for someone who's trying to maintain their brain health is the ketogenic diet. It's a really strict diet designed to make your body start burning fat, because you're no longer feeding your body the carbs for glucose. Your body then starts converting the stored fat into ketones, and your brain loves ketones. Your brain does much better on a ketogenic diet. Any neurodegenerative disease improves with a ketogenic diet.

Second, reduce stress.

Most people don't perceive that they have a lot of stress; they just think: *That's life.*

You need to take one of the stress tests on the internet. You can find what your *stress score* is, and this will help you get a better look at your stress. Then, cut things out of your life that are stressful, and find ways to manage your stress in a better way. Start your day off with a gratitude journal, a prayer and meditation, tai chi, or yoga. Anything like that helps with stress.

You need to optimize sleep, and that means getting an overnight sleep test. There are some free tests, where your doctor can send you home to sleep with an oxygen checker, to see if you have low oxygen at night, because that will affect your brain health. If you do, then you need to have a sleep study, and get treated for sleep apnea if you have it.

Exercise is critical. I talked earlier in the book about nitric oxide bursts. You can perform two-, three-, or four-minute bursts per day, and that helps tremendously. High-intensity interval training is also helpful. You must exercise to keep your brain healthy. Quality exercise reduces insulin levels, and insulin levels that are high in your brain affect your cells significantly.

Stimulate your brain. There are many programs online that you can use to test yourself; some brain health game programs will keep track of your score and your speed. Doing these exercises three times a week is great. Work the *New York Times* crossword puzzle or try *sudoku* – a Japanese number puzzle. Challenge your brain on a regular basis. Other strategies include learning something new, such as how to knit, play a musical instrument, or speak a new language. Including movement and a social component greatly enhance the benefit to brain health.

Then, you need to get your hormones balanced. If your adrenal glands aren't working properly and your hormone levels are off, you need to find a practitioner to get those fixed. That includes your thyroid. Do not just get a TSH; you need to get a full thyroid assessment with antibodies to make sure your thyroid is optimal.

Maintaining good GI health is vital: To maintain good GI health, you must first know if you have gut problems such as bacteria, yeast, or parasites. You can find that in a stool test. Then, maintain that health with prebiotics and probiotics, and eating fermented foods and other healthy foods for the GI tract.

You need to optimize lab levels for any lab level that is out of range. If you have a predisposition to dementia, you especially need to tighten up the range. I don't mean the lab ranges that come back from the lab. I mean the functional ranges that the functional medicine community uses. They have been really tightened up for dementia prevention. For example, we keep your insulin levels and your glucose levels really low, and we keep the inflammatory markers really tight. That helps maintain a healthy brain.

Supplementation is needed. If you need CoQ10, omega-3s, vitamins A, C, or D, you should be taking those supplements. That is what your practitioner will tell you. Here again, you have to go to a trained practitioner. You can't just go to your family GP. They do not know what vitamins and supplements you need. They don't have the time and they are not paid to do that, so go to someone who knows what they're doing.

Last of all, dental hygiene: It seems very odd to talk about dental hygiene with the brain and Alzheimer's, but on autopsies, brains have been found with the bacteria that causes gingivitis. They relate gingivitis and oral health to an increased rate of Alzheimer's. If you have gingivitis, you need to start doing coconut oil pulling every day. You need to brush and floss after every meal. You must be stringent with your oral health. Remember, prevention is about treating deficiencies and removing toxins.

If you're diagnosed with cognitive impairment, all of the same protocols that I just talked about apply. In addition, with the diagnosis of a mild cognitive impairment your healthcare practitioner may prescribe Aricept for a month. It's a drug for dementia. Newer drugs are coming out as well, such as Mamzarit. It's a combination drug, which is helpful for two of the holes in the roof. The entire protocol we've been discussing is essential, in addition to any drugs that may be prescribed to you.

One other thing: I want to talk about caregiving, because caring for someone with cognitive decline causes a cognitive decline in the caregiver. If you are caring for someone with cognitive decline, your risk just went way up even if you don't have the ApoE-4 gene. If you do have the gene, your risk of getting it has gone up because of the stress.

Caring enough for your spouse or partner to *prevent* cognitive decline will enhance life and improve quality of aging—and healthy aging. You have to start the process before cognitive issues start; you have to be proactive to have a good, healthy life. I think it is critical for people in their forties to begin addressing these issues.

It is never too late, even if you have full-blown Alzheimer's. It's never too late to start, even if you have a mild cognitive decline or you're on the drug. Doing everything I talked about here will help minimize the symptoms and give you a better quality of life.

Regarding healthcare, first, you must find a qualified functional medicine practitioner, preferably trained by Dr. Dale Bredesen in the ReCODE *(Reversing Cognitive Decline)* process. Hundreds of practitioners in the U.S. have been trained in the protocol, and I happen to be one of them.

Second, do not allow traditional medicine to give you a death sentence.

Do not go into your primary care provider, get a diagnosis of early dementia, and have them give you a drug and say: *See you in a year.*

People still think Alzheimer's is a death sentence, and they allow traditional medicine to encourage that thinking. It is not a death sentence. Get your genetic testing and book a consult with a practitioner who can interpret it and put you on a program, figure out what else is wrong, and help you turn your life around.

CHAPTER FIVE

Exploring Common Myths about Healthcare

STATINS

The general population has been brainwashed to think that high cholesterol is caused by what you eat. That is simply not true. Twenty to 25 percent of cholesterol in your body comes from diet, and studies have found that there's no correlation between eating red meat, animal fat, eggs, butter, cheese, sausage, bacon, and the like, and elevation of cholesterol. That's the number-one myth I'm going to try to dispel in this chapter. When the cholesterol intake goes down, your body compensates by making more cholesterol.

The number-two myth is that statin drugs will improve your heart health. Statin drugs are a multi-billion-dollar business in this country. A large percentage of the population — 17 percent of the U.S. population ages forty to fifty-nine and 48 percent of those seventy-five years and older — takes statin medications.

Statins decrease your levels of coenzyme Q10 (CoQ10), which is essential for energy level, quality of life, and longevity. CoQ10 is involved in cellular respiration and the production of ATP. It is used for energy production in every cell in your body. Your heart is the number one consumer of energy, and it demands the most energy. Reducing the energy supply can be pretty devastating. So, if you are on a statin and you are over age forty, you must take a supplement, like *ubiquinol*, which is a reduced form of CoQ10.

Cholesterol Benefits

Cholesterol is a sterol that plays a crucial role in forming cell membranes. Every cell in our body has cholesterol in its membranes. Without a cell membrane, we would have no cells — so you must have cholesterol for your body. I see patients who are so proud of their lowered cholesterol level.

They tell me, "It's down to 120!"

I just about have heart failure thinking: *Oh my gosh, these people are just subjecting themselves to a lack of cholesterol in their cells!*

Cholesterol is important for our lives. Our bodies do create 70–80 percent of our cholesterol, so only 20–25 percent comes from the diet. The body so tightly regulates cholesterol that if you eat less cholesterol, your body will simply produce more. Cholesterol is so important that your body is designed to create enough for vital functions.

Cholesterol is a precursor for making sex hormones. I find many of my patients are concerned about their sex hormones: women, with their estrogen and progesterone, and men, with their testosterone. If you don't have enough cholesterol, the first hormones to stop being produced are sex hormones. That's an important point to keep in mind. Cholesterol benefits your body in many ways. Without it, you would cease to exist.

Proper Lab Testing

High cholesterol is not a disease. High cholesterol is a symptom, so we must investigate what the underlying cause is. In functional medicine, we don't simply suppress the symptom by prescribing a statin drug for you. Instead, we look at the underlying cause of the elevated cholesterol if it's extremely elevated. When we order lab testing, we assess cholesterol and triglycerides, and, with respect to cholesterol, we specifically look at the LD(a) and LDL-p, the number of low-density lipoprotein particles. This lab assessment of the number of particles that we oxidize predicts higher risks for cardiovascular disease better than LDL cholesterol, blood pressure, age, smoking, and other factors. Most of the public does not know anything about LD(a) or LDL-p. Since it is a really good predictor of cardiovascular disease, when you get your labs, you should ask for your LD(a) and LDL-p.

Cardiovascular disease is prompted by inflammation; that is the root cause. With the Standard American Diet, and the high levels of sugar in the diet, inflammation is common. Other markers that you need to look for, when you're assessing cholesterol, is *C-Reactive Protein,* also known as CRP or hs-CRP. If it's elevated, then this indicates that the inflammatory response, which gives you an increased risk for cardiovascular events, is present. It's very predictive of your risk, more so than cholesterol and triglycerides. Many people don't know that, and the majority of practitioners do not order that test. It's a simple test to order. I order it for every patient.

Another marker is *homocysteine.* This is a naturally occurring amino acid that requires B_{12}, folate, and B_6 to function properly. Elevated homocysteine irritates the lining of the blood vessels, causing them to get hard and narrow. Increased levels of homocysteine also increase blood clotting, so it is beneficial to know your homocysteine level. The test is simple to order from any lab and will give you an idea of how inflamed you are.

Finally, good blood sugar testing should be done. Most people come in with just the glucose testing that their primary care doctor has done. Studies have consistently shown that glucose testing does not predict anything for the future; it is just telling you how much sugar you have on board from the last time you ate.

Studies consistently show the risk for heart attack more than doubles when blood sugar levels are elevated. If a patient is in the prediabetic range, they have a double risk for cardiovascular disease, compared to someone whose blood sugar is in the low nineties. So, we check a person's two- to three-month average by doing a hgA1C—*hemoglobin A1C*. We can also do tests for post-meal blood sugars. In fact, you can do post-meal blood sugars test yourself. If you do a forty-five minute to an hour blood-sugar check at home, with a home kit, and another one at two hours, the glucose numbers at one hour should be less than 140 mg/dL, and at two hours, less than 120 mg/dL. If they're not, you have an increased cardiovascular risk. With a blood sugar home testing kit, you can actually determine your increased cardiovascular risk.

People can go to a lab for these tests. In most instances, you can walk in and get a test; your insurance may not cover it, but it's worth the money, the investment in your health, to get the testing and know what your numbers are. You have to know your numbers.

A Functional Approach to Treating High Cholesterol

If you have elevated cholesterol, try to protect your heart. Diet and exercise are the number-one and number-two ways of protecting your heart. In your diet, to reduce cholesterol and triglycerides, you've got to avoid sugars, grains, and gluten. In a managed diet, when grains and sugars are cut, I've seen triglyceride levels drop several hundred points.

You also have to manage stress because stress contributes to cardiovascular disease.

There are many different tactics to reduce stress:

- Practicing forms of mindfulness
- Yoga
- Meditation
- Prayer
- Writing in a gratitude journal
- Exercise

Get plenty of animal-based omega-3 fats. Krill oil is inexpensive, and 500 milligrams per day can improve your cholesterol and triglycerides, and increase high-density lipoprotein (HDL) levels, which is what people refer to as the *good* cholesterol.

For cardiovascular health, you need restorative sleep. As we've already discussed, if you don't know if you have sleep apnea or some type of sleep disorder, a lot of home oxygen companies will let you take a monitor home and do an overnight test in your own bedroom. If you have some sleep apnea episodes, then that would indicate you need to get a sleep study.

Restorative sleep is important for many health reasons. Make it dark in your room. Keep the animals out of your bed. Use your bedroom only for sex and sleep. Make sure you do something quiet; no blue lights and no computer screens before you go to sleep. There are a lot of things you can do to make sure you get restorative sleep.

You need to make sure your gut health is good, and you can start by adding some live, fermented foods to your diet. That's an inexpensive and easy thing to do. Add some sauerkraut or kimchi—just a tablespoon or two a day is very good for your gut. In addition, take probiotics—they are really good for heart health.

Another thing to pay attention to is your oral hygiene. Oral hygiene is a large contributor to cardiovascular health. You need to floss after every meal. You should be using the protective process of coconut oil pulling: put some coconut oil in your mouth and swish it back and forth. You pull it between your teeth, back and forth, and continue for five to ten minutes, then spit it out. Don't swallow it, because it will be full of the bacteria you've just removed from your teeth and gums.

Exercise regularly. Do high-intensity interval training because it increases healing growth factor, and it will help you to lose weight. It increases your calorie burn for up to two hours after the exercise. Do the nitric oxide bursts that I referred to in a previous chapter; they will help relax the cardiovascular system. As we've already discussed, you can find Dr. Mercola's nitric oxide exercises online.

A functional approach to cardiovascular disease requires your attention to all of the factors mentioned here.

Reuters reported in 2014 that health regulators are adding a warning to labels of cholesterol-lowering drugs such as statins to say they may increase blood sugar and could cause memory loss. In closing this section, if you are on a statin drug, you really need to go see a functional practitioner and get your numbers—your lab results—and figure out what you really need to do, because you are at risk for developing diabetes and dementia by continuing to take statin drugs.

It's tough to change the thinking that has been perpetuated by the pharmaceutical companies, the thinking in which our primary care doctors have been trained. Statin sales are a whopping $140 billion per year. It's hard to change people's thinking when that much money is being made by one product. Just stop and think before you let a practitioner prescribe a statin drug for you. Remember a few of the things I've mentioned in this chapter.

GERD MEDICATION

The myth is that acid reflux is caused by too much hydrochloric acid in the stomach, and it must be suppressed. That is what most Americans believe, that they have to suppress acid in order to eradicate heartburn. But in fact, all of the studies have shown hydrochloric acid decreases as you get older. That's generally when you start getting heartburn. One cause of GERD is a decrease of hydrochloric acid in the stomach.

The mainstream, allopathic medicine approach is to take acid-suppressing drugs for as long as symptoms are present. People start taking them, and they take them for the rest of their lives because the root cause of reflux is never identified in treatment. Many pharmaceutical texts suggest over-the-counter GERD medications should not be used for more than two weeks, and prescribed *proton pump inhibitors* (PPI), less than a year. You should not take over-the-counter acid-suppressing medication for more than two weeks, either, but many in the population take them for their lifetime. If you are currently taking an antacid or a PPI, make sure that you consult with your prescribing practitioner before changing or stopping your dosage. Abruptly stopping this medication could result in severe symptoms.

The Benefits of Hydrochloric Acid and the Side Effects of Taking GERD Meds

Hydrochloric acid is a prerequisite for healthy digestion. If you don't have hydrochloric acid, you cannot break down and absorb nutrients. The acidity in your stomach is in a very narrow range. If you do not have enough hydrochloric acid, nutrients won't be absorbed, and you can end up with anemia, osteoporosis, cardiovascular disease, depression, anxiety, and insomnia. Most people cannot imagine how hydrochloric acid is related to, for instance, anxiety, depression, and insomnia. If you have enough hydrochloric acid, it breaks down proteins. Proteins are made of amino acids, and amino acids are the essential building blocks for neurotransmitters. Depression, anxiety, and sleep all have neurotransmitters involved.

If you do not have enough hydrochloric acid, or you are taking a drug that suppresses it, your proteins are going to escape digestion, due to a lack of the acid. This then triggers the production of peptins. Peptins are proteins that end up in the bloodstream, and the body reacts to them as if they were foreign invaders. You end up with what is called a *leaky gut.*

When these proteins leak out into your bloodstream, they get caught up in different tissues, such as the thyroid. They may pop over into the brain, and this can result in allergic reactions such as autoimmune disease. It's critical to get those proteins broken down so that they don't enter into the bloodstream at a larger size, and cause all of these autoimmune and allergic reactions.

In addition, if you have reduced acid, either because of age or due to taking a medication to inhibit acid, this will reduce the absorption of iron, B_{12}, folate, calcium, and zinc. Folate is critical for a healthy cardiovascular system, and the prevention of birth defects. If you can't absorb calcium, it affects your bones, teeth, and thousands of chemical reactions in your body. These all require calcium.

There are two types of acid-suppressors. They come in two basic varieties. Firstly, there are *histamine-receptor blockers,* which were developed to treat peptic ulcers, but are now available over the counter. They are Tagamet, Zantac, Pepcid, and Axid. Possible side effects of these drugs are that they interfere with metabolism of estradiol and testosterone and increase the risk of an *h. pylori* infection in your gut.

The other class of acid-suppressing drugs is *proton pump inhibitors,* or PPIs. They inhibit the proton pump in the stomach; specifically, the proton pumps in the cells in the lining of the gut. One of these pills can significantly decrease stomach acid for most of the day. Using PPIs can contribute to malnourishment because you're not breaking down the food that you eat and are unable to utilize the nutrients in the food. According to the inserts that come with the drug, possible side effects of long-term PPI use include increased risk of heart attacks, fractures, and kidney function failure. Cancers may also be related to it, as well as diarrhea, skin reactions, headaches, impotence, breast enlargement, and gout.

Overall, when stomach acid gets too low, you're susceptible to a wide range of serious disabilities. I refer to Dr. Jonathan Wright and Lane Leonard, PhD for the list of disabilities. *Why Stomach Acid Is Good for You,* by Jonathan Wright (Rowman & Littlefield Publishers, 2001) is an excellent book that you should buy and read. Many people think these symptoms are simply due to aging but these symptoms can also be from low acid levels.

According to Dr. Wright, some of the symptoms of low stomach acid are allergies, bronchial asthma in childhood, depression, bacterial overgrowth leading to heartburn, gas, constipation and diarrhea, pernicious anemia, stomach cancer, skin diseases including acne, dermatitis, and eczema, gall-bladder issues, rheumatoid arthritis, lupus, Graves' disease, ulcerative colitis, chronic hepatitis, osteoporosis, type 1 diabetes, and accelerated aging. Again, acid is our friend, and we need it to avoid these types of situations.

The Functional Approach to Treatment

Normally, when patients come in to see me, I don't have them stop their GERD medicine cold turkey. The majority of patients who come in and don't feel well are taking an acid reflux medication. Once I start treating them, they feel better, so I start tapering their reflux medication. We have them take an H2, which is a *histamine-receptor blocker* — such as Zantac — along with their PPI. After two to three weeks, we cut the PPI in half. After four to five weeks, we reduce it to taking it two-thirds of the time; taking the medication for two days, then skipping the third. Week six to seven, they're taking it every other day. Week eight to nine, once every three days; and weeks nine to ten, once a week. On week eleven or twelve, they stop. Then after two more weeks, they stop the histamine-receptor blocker that they're taking, as well.

That is the taper protocol, and you can do this with guidance from your practitioner, but you'll also need to do the three Rs that go along with it.

The first R is *reduce*. First, you need to reduce your high-carb diet. You have to eliminate artificial sweeteners, and sometimes, you may need to reduce some of your high fiber if you're taking a lot of high-fiber foods. If the diet change doesn't help, you need to check and see if you have an *h. pylori* infection, and then you need to treat it if so.

The second R is *replace*. Your practitioner can replace the stomach acid with a product with hydrochloric acid that has enzymes and protease in it.

And the last R is *restore*. Then you can take bitter herbs, which you can find over the counter, or apple cider vinegar, lemon juice, sauerkraut, or pickles. If you've had GERD and you're taking an inhibitor medication, you should supplement with B_{12}, folic acid, calcium, iron, and zinc. You should test your levels first, then follow the levels of lab tests as indicated. I don't normally recommend people supplement with calcium, but if you've been on GERD medicine, you need to do that for a while.

Most people who see me — once they change their diet — really do start eliminating their medication right away without me even initiating it. They feel better and they don't have any symptoms! Part of the *restore* is taking probiotics, fermented foods, small amounts of kefir or yogurt, sauerkraut, pickles, or bone broth. They all help the healing of the gut lining. Deglycyrrhizinated licorice (DGL) is often helpful as well.

If these measures don't help, you need to consult with a knowledgeable physician that may need to do a surgical procedure to repair the lower esophageal sphincter — the muscle that prevents stomach acid from getting pushed up into esophagus.

In closing, I am concerned about the millions of people who are taking this medication without knowing the FDA limitation of two weeks. It's not widely published, and the consumers are not educated. If you're taking a GERD medicine, you need to find a functional practitioner who can help you get off that — but first of all, figure out what the root cause of your problem is. You need someone who can do the testing, then help you with the tapering, the diet, and the supplements that you need to take.

SUNSCREEN AND VITAMIN D

The myth out there is that the sun will give you skin cancer, therefore you must use a sunscreen. That's the myth, and the problem with that is that we then end up with all of these people with vitamin D deficiencies.

You have to remember that as an ancient culture, we were running around with wolf skin over us, year-round, out in the sun, fully exposed. Genetically, we are predisposed to be able to tolerate the sun. In 1903, they started sunlight therapy again, after we became cultured and started being covered up from head to toe with long skirts and body covers. The sunlight therapy was discovered by Dr. August Rollier in 1903 in Switzerland. Of the 2,157 patients he treated, 1,746 completely recovered from tuberculosis. He started doing sunlight therapy because his girlfriend got TB.

For forty years, they treated TB in sanitariums. People were sent to sanitariums for good food and sun. They sat out in the sun, and that was the main treatment that they got. All those years, sunlight was used to treat skin problems, nervous system problems, musculoskeletal problems, and respiratory problems. Even eyes, ears, nose, and throat issues were treated with sunlight therapy.

As drugs have grown and the sunscreen industry has grown, sunlight has fallen to the wayside. Now, we are threatened and cautioned that we will get cancer if we're out there, and we have to put on lots of sunscreen. There, again, there comes a market, a billion-dollar industry, that has been created around sunscreen. My concern for the consumer is that, there again, they are not educated as to the benefits of vitamin D.

Benefits of the Sun

Again, we have to remember that we evolved hunting and foraging under the sun, with next to no clothing on. Ultraviolet-B waves from the sun help convert dehydrocholesterol on the skin into previtamin D_3.

If you use sunscreen all the time, if you use a Sun Protection Factor (SPF) over fifteen, you get no benefits from the sun. It is recommended that you go out in the sun without sunscreen, because of the absolute requirements for healthy living. This is taken from the Institute for Functional Medicine. They have a nice summary of vitamin D levels and the benefits of the sun which you can access by contacting an IFM-trained practitioner.

Let me just tell you the conditions that are associated with vitamin D levels below thirty nanograms per milliliter. Most people are hanging in between thirty and forty nanograms, and that is insufficient. Below thirty, you have a high risk of rickets, and a seventy-five percent greater risk of colon cancer. Around thirty, you also have increased loss of calcium from bones, which leads to osteoporosis, poor wound healing, increased muscle pain, increased joint and back pain, greater risk of depression, increased diabetes, increased schizophrenia, increased migraines, increased autoimmune, increased allergies, increased preeclampsia — which is a problem in pregnancy — and increased inflammation. This information again comes from the IFM.

At a suboptimal level of thirty to fifty nanograms, you have twice the risk of heart attack, increased incidences of high blood pressure, and three times the risk of multiple sclerosis.

Most practitioners will tell you, if your vitamin D level is between thirty and fifty, it is fine. I would not want to be *fine* and have those risks! From fifty to eighty nanograms, you have reduced your risk of cancer by fifty percent. You have a decreased risk of all solid cancers. Between eighty and one hundred, you have a slowing of cancer growths in patients with cancer. Over one hundred nanograms, you have an increased risk of toxic symptoms, such as hypercalcemia, which is too much calcium in the blood. There's tremendous risk to not having adequate vitamin D levels.

I always tell my patients, "Know your numbers."

You should know what your vitamin D number is.

Effects of Sunscreen

The danger of sunscreen—according to Dr. Joseph Mercola's book, *Dark Deception* (p. 120)—besides making you deficient in vitamin D, is that sunscreens may be making a huge contribution to the toxin load in your body.

There are dangerous chemicals found in most sunblocks, and I want to give you a short list of some of the chemicals:

- Para-aminobenzoic acid
- Avobenzone
- Cinoxate
- Dioxybenzone
- Homosalate

I'm not going to list all of them, but he lists fourteen different toxic chemicals that are found in sunscreen. So not only are you slathering sunscreen all over yourself and your poor children, head to toe, but you're exposing them and yourself to toxins. Plus, you are creating a vitamin D deficiency. You really need to consider eliminating sunscreen. I have not used sunscreen in a couple years. I have not gotten a sunburn, and I am very healthy. I think most people need to do that. A word of caution to those who are still using aerosol sunscreens: not only do you contaminate your own area but you may also be triggering reactions in the people surrounding you.

The Functional Approach to Treating Vitamin D Deficiency

Look at a food list for vitamin D, and try to incorporate some foods high in vitamin D.

I would prefer that people get enough vitamin D from food. However, most processed, refined foods that have vitamin D are enriched with vitamin D_2. Vitamin D_2 is not effective in your body, but they put that in because they can charge for it. It's a manufactured, artificial component. If you can't get it from food—you can eat a lot of fish and a few others, but there's not a lot—I generally recommend a vitamin D_3 supplement. You can get it as a liquid or a pill you take once a day, or in some places, you can get injections. I think you need to take Vitamin D on a regular basis.

The normal dosing for vitamin D depends on your blood level and your specific health conditions. For a blood level of less than 50 nanograms per milliliter, but higher than 30, I'd recommend about 2,000 to 3,000 International Units (IU) per day. For a level down to 20 or 30, I'd give 10,000 IU per day of vitamin D_3. What you take depends on your level. I don't want my patients to become toxic.

Also, start going out in the sun year-round. Go out on your lunch break, sit in a sunny spot, and get some sun on your arms, chest, and face. A red-headed person with fair skin may only tolerate ten minutes before they burn. A black-skinned person may not burn at all. Different skin types really take different levels of sun. Set a timer when you first start and progressively stay out longer. Don't get sunburned. The cause of melanoma is not the sun itself; it is getting sunburned over and over. When your children are in the water, they should have protective shirts and clothing that block out the ultraviolet rays. Just be really cautious when you first start. Get out there and get that natural exposure.

One other thing for both women and men: You should wear a hat after a brief exposure to protect your face. Your facial skin is very fragile. To avoid wrinkles long-term, as you get older, it's important to wear a hat to protect your face. If you're going to be out gardening or golfing all day, put a hat on.

Conclusion

In closing, I want people who have read this book to realize the amazing power of the human body to heal itself, once given the proper nutrients, exercise, and removal of toxins and bugs. Our bodies were designed to be healthy. If you are not healthy, then you need to look seriously at what kind of help you can get. The most important place to start is with a functional medicine practitioner who understands *root cause*.

If you're not feeling well, if you're not healthy, there is a root cause, and you need to figure out what it is so you can correct it and achieve a much better, healthier life.

Those of you who know that you just need to lose a little weight and you'll feel better, jump in and try one of the new diets we discussed. Eliminate the processed, refined foods. Start walking. Get a friend or a buddy who will do it with you. Often your spouse is an ideal partner to work with to start changing the way you eat, changing the way you exercise, and changing your life in baby steps.

If you do address everything that I talked about in this book for one full year, at the end of that year, your health will be so much better than when you started.

The hardest part is starting. Take that first step.

My final advice is this quote, attributed to Hippocrates:

> *Everyone has a physician inside him or her,*
> *we just have to help it in its work. The natural*
> *healing force within each one of us is the*
> *greatest force in getting well.*

Appendix

The elimination diet is an excellent way to give your body a rest from any possible inflammatory foods. For more about how this fits into your total health picture, see Chapter One's section on the Five Rs.

Week 1:

- Eat at least two servings of cooked, raw, or fermented vegetables and fruits per meal from the list provided below.

- Consume 2–3 cups of bone broth per day. Use it for vegetable soup if needed.

- Remove all caffeine, hydrogenated fats, and artificial sweeteners from your diet.

It is important to ensure adequate protein throughout this and all phases of detoxification. Avoid charbroiled meats.

Week 2:

- Eat at least two servings of cooked, raw, or fermented vegetables per meal from the list provided below.

- Continue bone broth.

- Remove all sugar and fruit juice (excluding cranberry juice) from your diet.

    Reaction note: the first several days after eliminating sugar can result in symptoms of brain fog or hangover as your body readjusts to functioning without sugar's quick energy. This will pass after a few days, depending on how sugar-reliant your body is.

Week 3:

- Eat at least three servings of vegetables per meal using cooked, raw, or fermented vegetables from the list provided. Raw or fermented vegetables should make up to ¼ - ½ cup of your total amount, one to three times per day with meal.

- Continue bone broth.

- Remove all gluten and corn from your diet.

Week 4:

- Eat at least four servings of vegetables per meal using cooked and raw, fermented vegetables from the list provided. Raw, fermented vegetables should make up ¼–½ cup, one to three times per day with meal (counts as above vegetable servings).

- Continue bone broth.

- Remove all grains, potatoes, soy, dairy, and alcohol.

Week 5:

- Eat at least four servings of vegetables per meal using cooked and raw, fermented vegetables from the list provided. Raw or fermented vegetables: ¼ - ½ cup, one to three times per day with meal (counts as above vegetable servings).

- Continue bone broth.

- Remove all eggs, tomatoes, shellfish, and legumes (including peanuts, though green beans are ok).

Eat organic, pasture-raised, wild-caught meats, and organic vegetables whenever possible.

The following vegetables and fruit support Phase II Detoxification. In the initial weeks of your elimination diet, stick to the leafy green options, limiting your intake of starchier vegetables, and limiting your intake of fruits to one serving per day:

- Alfalfa sprouts
- Artichokes
- Asparagus
- Avocado
- Beets
- Beet greens
- Berries: blueberries, raspberries, strawberries
- Bok choy
- Broccoli
- Brussels sprouts
- Cabbage
- Carrot
- Cauliflower
- Celery
- Chard
- Cherries
- Collards
- Cucumbers
- Dandelion greens
- Garlic
- Grapefruit
- Kale
- Leeks
- Mustard greens
- Onion
- Orange
- Parsnips
- Pumpkin

- Red peppers
- Salad greens
- Sauerkraut
- Spinach
- Squash
- String beans
- Sweet potatoes
- Turnips
- Zucchini

Next Steps

I'm always happy to travel to talk to groups about health. Some of my favorite topics are stress hormones, belly fat, thyroid issues, and restoring and preventing cognitive decline. I can talk pretty well about anything that a group would like, so I'm always open to suggestions.

I am available for a free ten-minute consultation to see if there is anything I might be able to help you with. Go on my website, NewHealthMontana.com, and schedule a ten-minute appointment. I use Telemedicine for remote work with clients. If you are in the Missoula, Montana area, just call my office at 406-721-2537. Schedule an introductory visit to discuss your symptoms and how we can start a program for you.

Because you have read the book, you would qualify for a reduced initial consultation fee. You know a lot more information than the average person, so it would take me less time to explain everything. There's always a special fee if you've read the book or gone to one of my lectures.

About the Author

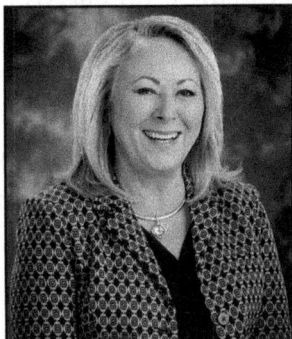

Donna Kay Jennings is an Advanced Practice Registered Nurse. Kay owns and operates several specialized healthcare facilities in Montana. She finds her passion in treating patients with a functional medicine approach.

Kay has a bachelor's degree and a master's of science in nursing, a master's degree in healthcare administration, and is a board-certified Psychiatric Mental Health Nurse Practitioner. She was a Vietnam-era captain in the U.S. Army Nurse Corps. She has post-graduate training in obesity medicine, as well as a Master Psychopharmacology Certification. In addition, Kay is Kresser Institute Adapt Trained (Level 1) and has completed the Institute of Functional Medicine coursework.

Over the years, Kay has lectured to the general public on many topics, such as stress hormones, thyroid, obesity, and the brain. She is also a frequent writer of health articles for the local newspapers and magazines in Montana.

In her spare time, Kay loves to travel, try new recipes, and paint. In addition, she rescues greyhounds. She also loves to entertain her extended family and friends.

Kay's website is NewHealthMontana.com. The phone number to reach her is 406-721-2537.

www.ingramcontent.com/pod-product-compliance
Lightning Source LLC
Chambersburg PA
CBHW070801290326
41931CB00011BA/2101